Alternative Health Options

&

Forty Years of MS

by Charles (Tip) Tiffany

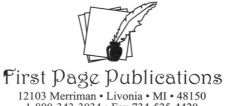

First Page Publications
12103 Merriman • Livonia • MI • 48150
1-800-343-3034 • Fax 734-525-4420
www.firstpagepublications.com

First Page Publications
12103 Merriman Road
Livonia, MI 48150
800-343-3034
www.firstpagepublications.com

Cover Image

Photo Researchers Picture Number: SB1530"Credit: Susumu Nishinaga / Photo Researchers, Inc."Description: Blood vessels. Colored scanning electron micrograph (SEM) of a resin cast of blood vessels in connective tissue. The fine network of smaller vessels branching off from the main vessel infiltrates the tissue, supplying it with blood. Gases and nutrients are exchanged between the blood and surrounding tissues through the permeable walls of capillaries, the smallest of blood vessels. Connective tissues provide structural support and cohesion throughout the body. The cast was made by injecting resin into the blood vessels, followed by chemical digestion of the surrounding tissues. Magnification: x27 at 6x7cm size.
Link: "http://db2.photoresearchers.com/search/SB1530"
Contact info:"Photo Researchers, Inc."60 East 56th Street, 6th Floor"New York, NY 10022"Tel: 212-758-3420"Fax: 212-355-0731
"http://www.photoresearchers.com"info@photoresearchers.com"

Library of Congress Cataloging-in-Publication Data

Tiffany, Charles, 1938-
 Alternative health options & forty years of MS / by Charles (Tip) Tiffany.
    p. cm.
 Includes bibliographical references.
 ISBN 1-928623-16-6
 1. Multiple sclerosis—Alternative treatment. I. Title: Alternative health options and forty years of MS. II. Title.
 RC377.T54 2004
 616.8'3406—dc22
        2004026111

Dedication

This book is dedicated to my wife, Hilary, who has stood beside me and been my rock for many years. Being a caregiver for someone who has MS in addition to working a full-time job is a tremendous responsibility. I don't always show my appreciation and thank her for all she does. I know there are things she would rather be doing. The number of everyday jobs I am physically able to do has deteriorated over the last fifteen years and my short-term memory does not always keep up with the tasks I can accomplish.

I would also like to thank all the kind people out there. Hardly a day goes by that someone does not offer assistance when I go out with my walker or use my wheelchair. Many polite children will wait and hold a door. Parents should be proud when their children do something like that without having to be asked.

I want to compliment those people who have an open mind and are willing to read about alternative options. Many people believe without question what their doctors tell them. We are a generation of people who put a lot of faith and trust in their medical professionals. This book is not intended to destroy that concept, but to question it.

Table of Contents

Chapter 15

Introduction

Are you curious about what alternatives there are to mainstream medicine? Do you want to discover new ways to increase the quality of your health? Are you seeking an alternative?

My purpose in writing this book is to share my experiences with you and discuss some alternatives to conventional medicine which could increase your quality of health and life in general. People can reduce the effects of symptoms of disease through the approaches outlined in these pages.

Being in good health is a blessing and special care should be taken to maintain it. The old adage about an ounce of prevention being worth a pound of cure is good advice. It is much harder to repair than it is to prevent. Life is not always fair and the possibility of acquiring a disabling sickness is real.

What is the difference between allopathic and holistic medicine? Allopathic treats the symptoms through the prescription of drugs, whereas holistic treats the cause by inducing the body to heal itself. Simply put, holistic medicine is a more natural approach which does not rely on synthetic remedies. In our society, allopathic medicine seems to be more widely accepted.

When allopathic doctors say there is nothing else they can do, people tend to search for alternatives on their own. Mainstream medical professionals generally do not like to consider alternative treatments. That does not mean that some of these remedies do not work.

Many patients try unproven remedies without telling their doctors and others blindly follow ultra-conservative medical ideas. There is a balance: a patient trying alternative medicine does need the allopathic experience of a trained professional to monitor treatments. I have found benefits to both allopathic and homeopathic practices. People who have only one doctor are limiting themselves. I recommend seeking medical advice from a number of doctors. This will give you well-rounded medical care. Carefully consider advice from any doctor; the bottom line is whether or not treatments are working for you personally.

This book is particularly aimed at helping patients with multiple sclerosis. There are non-traditional treatments and supplements that can help patients handle their problems. I believe MS can be controlled. People with MS live it 24/7. Millions of dollars are spent on research trying to find a cure. Are we just to wait until they come up with a proven therapy? I am not one to sit back and wait.

The treatments and information described in this book are not intended to take the place of medical care. They are only options offered to you as a guide for your own exploration and for the discovery of alternative methods that may help improve your health.

CHAPTER 1
Multiple Sclerosis

This chapter explains MS, its symptoms, diagnosis, possible causes, and treatment options. It also explains the four levels of MS. Some of the material in this chapter is from an article by Ashton F. Embry, Ph.D. This complete article can be viewed at http://www.serafin.ch/embrye.htm.

Definition

Multiple sclerosis (MS) is an autoimmune disease in which patches of myelin in the eyes, brain, and spinal cord are damaged or destroyed. The myelin sheath is the multiple layers of insulation that cover the nerve fibers. This degeneration is caused by the entry of immune cells (e.g. T-cells, B-cells, and macrophages) into the central nervous system (CNS) through the walls of the cells. Damage to the blood-brain barrier (BBB) allows passage of components that are toxic to the myelin in the cerebral spinal fluid. When this occurs, impulses are not conducted properly. The covered protection of the nerve fibers by the myelin sheath allows electrical impulses to be conducted along the nerve fibers.

MS is a crippling disease but not a fatal one. Life expectancy for MS patients is only six or seven years less than the general population. Death most often occurs through normal causes like cancer, heart disease, or stroke. Death caused by a MS lesion to the brain is extremely rare.

 MS is a disease that involves excessive immune system activity, which is why most medical professionals profess that it is not good to build the immune system. The brain influences production of hormones that may affect the immune system, while the immune system secretes chemicals called cytokines. These cytokines influence nerve cell activity, which release chemicals called neurotransmitters. This affects the way the brain sends signals to the muscles.

At the present time, the medical profession does not know what causes this disease. Experts think there is a genetic predisposition for MS. The chance of acquiring MS is about 0.003–0.005 percent, roughly one or two people in every one hundred thousand.

Symptoms often vary from person to person. Most patients have heat intolerance, which can cause a temporary increase in fatigue or loss of coordination. When the body is cooled off, these symptoms may seem to disappear. Some patients may suffer from problems with balance, blurred vision, numbness, pain, and weakness. These symptoms generally become apparent in young adults between the ages of twenty to thirty-five.

It is very important to adhere to a good diet, ask for help, know your limits, listen to your body, plan a strategy to fight fatigue, rest when you tire, and talk to your doctor to explain your concerns. The disease is a difficult one to put into remission. It is a good idea to keep a journal of your symptoms. Not only will this be important should you have the need to apply for social security disability benefits, it will help you stay organized and know your symptoms better.

Persons with MS (PWMS) could possibly benefit from a paradigm shift. There are many choices that may be outside the scope of you or your doctor. After all, life is all about choices.

Diagnosis

Tests to diagnose MS include: the flicker-fusion and enhanced flicker-fusion test, magnetic resonance imaging (MRI), balance testing, red-cell mobility, spinal taps, and symptom-recurrence records. Serial Gadolinium-Magnetic Resonance Imaging (Gd-MRI) is a test for documenting the efficacy of treatments.

An article published in the *Annals of Neurology*, July 2002; 52(1): 47-53 titled "Application of the New McDonald Criteria to Patients With Clinically Isolated Syndromes Suggestive of Multiple Sclerosis," tells of a new diagnostic method using magnetic resonance imaging, along with diagnostic methods to test persons with just one episode of demyelination. This test was found to increase the diagnostic accuracy rate by as much as seventy-five percent. This article can be found at http://newfirstsearch.oclc.org/WebZ/FSFETCH?fetchtype=fullrecord:sessionid =sp05sw01-39234-djcxh31.

At this time, there is no cure and diagnosis is difficult because the symptoms are similar to that of other maladies. The worse thing you can do, if you are diagnosed with MS, is to do nothing at all. I believe a healing process can improve your health and give a degree of symptom relief.

The Four Types of MS

Type 1 RRMS:

Relapsing-remitting multiple sclerosis (RRMS) is the mildest form. With this type, symptoms will come and go. Early symptoms can be cold hands and feet, confusion, coordination difficulty, cramping, difficulty sleeping, bruising easily, joint pain, loss of energy, memory loss, muscle aching, nervousness, numbness in extremities, periodic fatigue, sensitivity to heat, temporarily blurred vision, and temperature fluctuations. It is a good idea to do treatment and make life style changes to prevent RRMS from slipping to SPMS.

Type 2 SPMS:

Secondary progressive multiple sclerosis (SPMS) is the next step where the severity of these symptoms is increased and the duration is extended and may not go away at all. In this type, incontinence and under or overactive bladder are common, caused by an interruption of the brain's message to the bladder.

Type 3 PPMS:

Primary progressive multiple sclerosis (PPMS) is an advanced stage of MS where the symptoms never go away. The PPMS person may be wheelchair bound and need assistance on a full-time basis. Double vision, jerky eye movement, loss of bowel or bladder control, loss of sensory feelings, loss of sight, loss of strength and mobility, nystagmus, paralysis, reflex impairment, and vertigo are common. Persons with PPMS can be stabilized for short periods of time.

Type 4 CPMS:

Chronic progressive multiple sclerosis (CPMS) is the most severe form of MS where the person's symptoms worsen progressively until they become bed-bound.

Possible Causes

There are many theories, but the root cause of MS is still a mystery and chances are there is no single cause. Some very basic assumptions are logical though. The first is that a person's genetic make-up has to be predisposed to being susceptible to MS. This theory is a little perplexing because one twin or sibling may have MS without the other being affected by it. It is not been proven to be hereditary or passed from one spouse to another, although increased risks to children have been noted.

MS is not believed to be contagious. Women are more likely to acquire MS than men by two to one. People who drank cow's milk as children were found to be more susceptible as adults. The incidence of MS at the Equator and North Pole is very low. The ratio of incidence of MS from coastal areas to farming areas is one to four.

There are hypothetical sources that tend to make adults more susceptible to acquiring MS. Some of the unproven theories are: low levels of cortisone, dopamine, histamine, vitamins B and D, high fat diets rich in gluten, dairy, and heavy metals including mercury, infection, and toxins. A deficiency in vitamin B6 and vitamin B12 may be associated with MS. Another theory relates to the use of sugar and aspartame contained in products marketed as NutraSweet®, Equal®, and Spoonful. If the temperature of aspartame exceeds eighty-six degrees Fahrenheit, the wood alcohol in aspartame converts to formaldehyde and then to formic acid (the poison found in the sting of fire ants) that in turn causes metabolic acidosis. The methanol toxicity mimics multiple sclerosis, but it is deadly. A relationship to measles and Epstein-Barr viruses has also been noted. MS is more prevalent in areas where selenium levels are low in the soil. Low copper levels are associated with defects in myelination.

There is a strong correlation to MS and diets high in animal fat, essential fatty acids or linoleic acid. A diet low in saturated fats, maintained over a long period of time, tends to retard MS. Allergy and food sensitivities may cause flare-ups. Cocoa, cola, coffee, milk, mold, fungi, mercury amalgam toxicity, and chocolate ingestion are all possible triggers. These food allergens can be identified by an Enzyme-linked Immunosorbent Assay (ELISA) test. Skin tests are a poor second choice because they have many limitations. All food allergens must be removed from your diet, as these are harmful to your BBB; while waiting to find these answers, it would be wise to stop eating all dairy products, gluten products, and eggs.

Prevention Treatments

There are many treatments available to help cope with MS. Conventional medical treatments are intended to lengthen the intervals between exacerbations. These treatments have related risks for possible side effects. If the treatment is started late in the duration of the disease, a reduction in the frequency of exacerbations or flare-ups is possible. Doctors who specialize in MS use one or a combination of six treatments. These choices were originally called the "ABC's"; that is Avonex®, Betaseron®, Copaxone®, and recently added are Antegren®, Novantrone, and Rebif®. People with heart problems, seizure, or suicidal ideation history need to be cautious when using these treatments. These drugs do not treat the underlying cause of the disease and have the potential for causing dangerous side effects. That is true for most treatments. The question is whether or not the discomfort is worth the gain, and it should be seriously discussed with your health care provider.

Treatments in General

Many PWMS don't take much medication. They may use Tylenol® and a few vitamins or mineral supplements. There has been always a controversy between allopathic (drugs) and homeopathic medicines (substances to help support the body's natural defenses to treat disease).

Drugs used to treat exacerbations may be taken orally (Dexamethasone or Prednisone) or intravenously (Methylprednisolone or Solumedrol). Drugs sometimes used to slow progression include Azathioprine, Cyclophosphamide, and Methotrexate.

With drugs, sometimes the cure is worse than the disease. Studies show a 40 percent decline in progression in approximately 30 percent of those using the allopathic approach. The present treatments are an attempt to slow the progression of the disease. IV Solumedrol has been found effective in stopping many MS exacerbations. Some of the drugs being used for fatigue are Amantadine and Provigil®. Drugs used for treating MS symptoms can be found at http://www.ms-doctors.org/medresource.shtml.

Almost every drug has potentially significant side effects. One medication alone will surely not win the battle against this disease. The patient has to be the one to decide whether or not to take the risk.

Case studies have been made of beneficial supplementation of an IV injection of 100 mg of nicotinic acid and 60 mg of thiamine (vitamin B1) in 10 cc solutions. B12 can be injected daily for a week with 1000 mg. Persons with adequate B12 respond well to treatments of adrenocorticotropic hormone (ACTH) that produce temporary remission. Years ago, this was the treatment of choice. Histamine has beneficial and therapeutic use for many diseases, including MS. The treatment of using procarin patches, which contain caffeine and histamine, might explain their benefit for some people. The combination of calcium and vitamin D may help suppress the disease. Tests have been made which show taking a vitamin D supplement for six months results in a remission and suppression of the immune system response that produces MS symptoms. Also noted was a decrease in interleuken-2 related to cells that induce MS. Excess vitamin D can be toxic.

Supplementation with linoleic acid, flaxseed oil, safflower oil, tryptophan, D-phenylalanine (DPA), and transcutaneous electrical nerve stimulation (TENS) may be beneficial.

The combination of calcium and magnesium is important in the development, structure, and stability of the myelin. Studies have shown an increase in MS in the intake of polyunsaturated fatty acids. Persons taking additional Omega-3 fatty acids (fish oils) may require additional vitamin E to prevent membrane peroxidation and cellular damage. It also significantly decreases platelet adhesiveness that inhibits the blood flow through the BBB.

The critical process in MS is the breakdown of the BBB that is necessary for MS to develop. Factors affecting the BBB include altitude, bacteria, diet, heat, heavy metals, hypertension, pollution, radiation, sanitation, sunlight, temperature, toxins, trauma, and viral infections. The Mayo Clinic has discovered a degradative enzyme called Myelencephalon Specific Protease (MSP) that could possibly block the process of tissue damage. This is very new, but it has real therapeutic potential and could stop the demyelination that occurs in MS patients. The Mayo Clinic has also done studies which show that having high levels of cytokines may help prevent nerve cells from damage.

List of Possible Treatments

If you are newly diagnosed, the doctor is likely to say there is no cure. True, there is no cure. Nothing approved by the FDA can prevent deterioration or make you better. You must take responsibility for your own life. The following is a list of available treatments. Ask your medical practitioner about them and ask for advice, but the final decision is yours.

- ACTH (Adrenocorticotropic Hormone)
- AMP (Adenosine Monophosphate)
- Antegren® (Natalizumab)
- ATP (Adenosine Triphosphate)
- Avonex® (interferon beta-1a)
- Betaseron® (interferon beta-1b)
- CamPath® (Alemtuzumab)
- Copaxone® (Glatiramer acetate)
- Depomedrol® (cortisone)
- Histamine
- LDN (Low Dose Naltrexone)
- Lipitor® (atorvastatin calcium)
- Novantrone (mitoxantrone hydrochloride)
- Prednosolone
- Prednisone (deltacortisone)
- Procarin patches (histamine and caffeine)
- QED (Quantum Electro Dynamics)
- Rebif® (interferon beta-1a)
- Solumedrol (Methylprednisolone)
- Stem cell (cell transplants)
- Swank diet (food regiment)
- 4-AP (4-aminopyridine)
- Natural approach

Furthermore, there is treatment of mitoxantrone combined with methylprednisolone that has shown some promise using the expanded disability status scale (EDSS).

ACTH (Adrenocorticotrophic Hormone) is a natural hormone produced by the anterior pituitary gland located at the base of the brain between the eyes. The adrenal glands can be tested for response to see if they are producing ACTH. It has been used to treat flares of MS, usually with positive results. ACTH is a cortisone-like steroid that can decrease inflammation and immune response. If the body does not have enough hormones like estrogen and testerone, possible side effects are an acceleration of the aging process and osteoporosis, both of which are common when steroids are used. Some physicians recommend use of vitamin D and calcium during use of steroids to decrease these side effects.

AMP (Adenosine Monophosphate) can either be administered with injection intramuscularly (IM) or on the skin. It can be mixed with histamine and caffeine in the form of a cream. AMP converts to Adenosine Triphosphate (ATP), which is a neurotransmitter and produces a number of coenzymes. Symptom improvement can include steadier balance, increased bladder control, and muscle strength. A prescription is needed for the IM type.

Antegren® (Natalizumab) is a new treatment which shows promising results for both Chron's Disease and MS. It is an Alpha-4 integrin inhibitor given by intravenous infusion every four weeks for six months. Tests show decreases in new lesion formation and reductions in the number of relapses. This antigen-specific immune therapy attacks the immune T-cells that attack the myelin. Possible side effects can be asthenia, back pain, fever, gastroenteritis, headache, rash, urinary tract infections, and urinary urgency. It is not a drug to be used on its own but in combination with others.

ATP (Adenosine Triphosphate) is a critical molecule in the cells of the body and is necessary for life. It helps build muscles, produce energy, and stimulate nerves. ATP in the cells works to remove one of the phosphate-oxygen groups leaving Adenosine Diphosphate (ADP), which is recycled in the mitochondria to once again become ATP. ATP transports substances across cell membranes and is used in conjunction with enzymes to bond certain molecules. Certain enzymes are involved in the formation and use of ATP. New sources of glucose are being developed that will be used to help create it.

Avonex® (interferon beta-1a) is for patients with RRMS and intended to slow the accumulation of physical disability and decrease the frequency of exacerbations. The FDA approved it in 1996. It is an injection given IM once a week, which has caused more patients to use Avonex. Tests have shown modest improvements in memory and other functions over a placebo. Possible side effects can include abdominal pain, asthenia, chest pain, chills, depression, fever, flu-like symptoms, headache, hypersensitivity, infection, injection site reactions, malaise, menstrual irregularities, muscle aches, ovarian cysts, pain, possible seizures, and suicidal ideation. Tests monitoring blood, white blood cell count, platelet count and liver function should be performed under a doctor's supervision. Medicare will cover Avonex when it is given in a doctor's office or hospital outpatient setting. Medicare will not cover Betaseron, Copaxone, or Rebif under any circumstances.

Betaseron® (interferon beta-1b) was the first of the "ABC" treatments on the market. It is intended for RRMS patients to increase the duration of remissions. Approved in 1993 by the FDA, the initial demand for a MS treatment was so great a lottery was set up as a fair sequence of dispersion. It is a purified, sterile, lyophilized protein product injected subcutaneous (SC) every other day. The dosage should be gradually increased as the body's tolerance builds. Liver tests and glucose levels should be checked while taking this treatment. Possible side effects include anxiety, chills, confusion, depression, dyspnoea, eating disorders, flu-like symptoms, fatigue, fever, guilt, indecisiveness, injection-site reactions, irritability, leukopenia, low self-esteem, lower white blood cell count, menstrual disorders, muscle aches, myalgia, necrosis, pain, palpitations, poor concentration, skin redness, shortness of breath, sleeping disorders, sweating, swelling, and suicidal tendencies.

CamPath® (Alemtuzumab) is an antineoplastic therapy used for treatment of B-Chronic Lymphocytic Leukemia (B-CLL). Single doses more than 30 mg daily or 90 mg weekly should not be used. Because of possible dangerous side effects, professionals should carefully monitor use of this drug.

Copaxone® (Glatiramer acetate for injection) is for patients with RRMS and was approved for use in 1995. Tests show it lengthens the intervals of remission. It is an injection given SC just under the skin daily and should not be administered intravenously. Possible side effects can include abdominal pain, anxiety, arthralgia, asthenia, chest pain, depression, dizziness, dyspnoea, fecal incontinence, flushing, headache, hypertonia, incontinence, infection, injection site reactions, nausea, pain, tremor, unintended pregnancy, urinary frequency, urinary tract infections, vasodilatation, vomiting, and urticaria. Copaxone at present has a pre-filled syringe for faster, easier injections. An oral dosage of Copaxone is presently being tested for treatment and will be approaching the FDA for approval. This is still in the early stages and will most likely not be on the market for a couple years following the publication of this book.

Depomedrol® is a drug I have found beneficial. This is administered by an injection into the hip. It is a steroid, and its use seems to calm symptoms.

Short-term use of steroids—about two weeks—should not caused undue concern, but long-term continuous use is apt to cause complications. Steroids can cause major nutrient losses of calcium and phosphorus contributing to adrenal exhaustion, a weakened immune system, and depression.

I have received two different medical opinions about safe time limits for its use. One doctor believes using it every six weeks is safe. The second used it on a ten-day basis for a severely disabled MS patient.

There have been no side effects in my case. I have received short-term temporary relief from symptoms with an injection of forty units of Depomedrol. I also use this as a pro-active maintenance therapy on a six-week basis during stressful times.

Histamine is a hormone/chemical transmitter in immune responses regulating allergic reactions and stomach acid production. Histamine is present in the body and when released in cells it causes vasodilatation and an increase in the permeability of blood vessel walls. Side effects can include wheezing and difficultly breathing. It should not be used for people with asthma.

LDN (Low Dose Naltrexone) is fairly new and non-toxic drug that can be taken nightly in capsule form with a prescription. Trials show positive results of ceasing MS progression in almost all patients. However, these trials are not scientific and considered anecdotal. Approximately two thirds of patients taking LDN notice symptom improvement within the first few days such as better ambulation and reduction in both spasticity and fatigue. This drug seems to cause a restoration of endorphin levels, improving energy.

Lipitor® (atorvastatin) is a commonly used cholesterol drug that influences the immune system. It can have an effect on reversing paralysis. Oral treatment of Lipitor could possibly prevent the induction of pro-inflammatory cytokines and induce secretion of anti-inflammatory cytokines. Lipitor could help insulin-dependant diabetes, melitis, multiple sclerosis, and rheumatoid arthritis.

Novantrone (mitoxantrone hydrochloride for injection concentrate) is used to reduce relapses, stabilize the disability, and decrease the number of new lesions. This is an anti-cancer drug and is being used on RRMS, SPMS, PPMS, but not CPMS patients. It is injected into a vein in the hand or arm. It has been shown effective in slowing the progression of disability in some patients. This is not suitable for all MS patients and should be discussed with your doctor due to risks. Persons with heart problems, liver disease, certain blood disorders, and a low number of white blood cells should not take Novantrone. Women should not become pregnant or breast-feed on this medication. Treatment varies from patient to patient. This treatment can be taken once every three months in the form of a five to fifteen minute IV infusion. It can be an IV infusion every month of 8 mg/m2 for one year. With this treatment, studies have shown that deterioration stopped and improvement was noted in patients with a rapidly deteriorating disease profile. The number of total lifetime doses allowable is limited and periodic testing is required. Possible side effects are bladder infections, hair thinning, loss of menstrual periods, lower white blood cell count, lower platelet count, mouth sores, and nausea. Because of the dark blue color of Novantrone, it may cause your urine to be blue-green and the white parts of your eyes may get slightly blue. Regular testing of the heart is required.

Prednisolone is a synthetic adrenal corticosteroid that has potent anti-inflammatory properties. It is used to treat a wide variety of conditions, particularly pertaining to the eyes and nose. It can be an oral tablet, topical cream, or gel.

Prednisone (deltacortisone) is an oral synthetic corticosteroid. It is used for suppressing the immune system and inflammation. It is converted in the liver to become prednisolone in patients whose adrenal glands are unable to produce enough amounts of cortisol.

Procarin patches are still considered experimental and must be bought at a compounding pharmacy with a prescription. Procarin is composed of FDA-approved products that are compounded in a gel or cream. This is then applied to the skin and covered with a patch to allow absorption. The primary components are histamine and caffeine. Some testimonials are encouraging.

QED (Quantum electro dynamics) is a homeopathic biofeedback system done on a Quantum Xrroid Conciousness Interface (QXCI) machine, an energic medical device. It is a fast, safe, non-invasive, and effective approach to healing. Sophisticated biofeedback software scans and corrects many problems by sending healing frequency waves to all parts of the body. This is a completely different approach to healing than western medicine offers. It helps remove the stressors— root causes of disease—and goes right to the base cells that are the cause of the problem. This is accomplished by the use of electrical bands applied around the ankles, forehead, and wrists that are connected to a PC with software through a converter box.

Rebif® (interferon beta-1a) is another new drug on the market. Similar to Avonex, in that it is an interferon, it is given subcutaneous three days a week and is not to be taken two days in a row. Some studies have shown better results with this therapy. It has been shown to slow the disability of MS and reduce relapses and the number and volume of lesions in the brain. Potential side effects are allergic reactions, anxiety, blood problems, depression, injection-site reactions, liver problems, pain, redness, risk to pregnancy, swelling, and thyroid problems.

Solumedrol (Methylprednisolone) is used to treat flares of MS. It is used with allergic reactions, asthma, collagen vascular diseases (e.g. Lupus), gastrointestinal diseases (ulcerative colitis and Chron's disease), and some lung diseases. Suggested use is of 1000 mg for seven days plus an oral dosage of decreasing strength for a tapering off period. This treatment is based on clinical practice, not research. Steroids normally accelerate the aging process and can cause cataracts, diabetes, muscle atrophy, osteoporosis, skin blemishes (temporary), and weight gain.

Stem cells are a promising form of treatment. There is a big political debate over their government funding. The question of ethics regarding the morality of using embryonic stem cells for research and treatment is being contested. Sixty percent of Americans support this research. This type of treatment could greatly benefit Alzheimer's, arthritis, diabetes, heart failure, MS, and Parkinson's. Stem cells can morph into any of the two hundred cell types of body tissue. Once in the body, the cell can divide and multiply indefinitely. It can also assist the development of different cell types.

There are four types of stem cells: adult, embryonic, fetal, and umbilical. Much of the controversy is over the embryonic type, as it is taken from a group of cells called a blastocyst that has not yet attached itself to the womb. This group of cells, after attachment, can become a human. These cells are totipotent and capable of developing into any type of mature cell. Most of these cells are produced in a fertility clinic where they are created by egg fertilization. The healthy cells can then be implanted in a uterus. This type of stem cell can be frozen and used at a later time. At present, as many as three hundred thousand stem cells are discarded as waste yearly. Adult stem cells are multipotent and limited to the type of cells they can produce. Adult stem cells are taken from specific tissue, such as blood, bone marrow, and skin. This type of stem cell is presently in trials in certain hospitals and other facilities in the United States, mostly for cancer treatment, but also on MS patients. The fetal type of stem cell is collected from an aborted fetus. Umbilical stem cells are drawn from the blood in the umbilical cord of a newborn baby. These stem cells are pluripotent and can give rise to most human tissues.

Only a few treatments have been done with stem cells. Hopefully this method will gain funding by the government, which will accelerate the possible treatment of many diseases. Stem cell transplantation studies need to be done to overcome the problem of immune rejection. Deoxyribonucleic acid (DNA) is part of a person's genes and unique to each individual, like a fingerprint.

Studies are being done in patients with severe MS using high-dose immune-suppression followed by autologous stem cell transplantation (donated by the patient).

The Swank Diet found in *The Multiple Sclerosis Diet Book* by Roy Swank, M.D., Ph.D. and Barbara Dugan has been proven beneficial, as it is low in saturated fats. Most people who stick to this diet find their symptoms improve. The four thousand patients monitored by Dr. Swank all noted improvements. It takes a lot of effort; things to avoid are: margarine, shortening, hydrogenated oils, red meat, dairy, alcohol, yogurt, cheese, and saturated fats.

4-AP (4-aminopyridine) is a drug called fampridine that is a nerve conduction-enhancing compound that has been proven to restore some neurological benefit to people with demyelinating CNS disorders. It acts on axons as a potassium-channel blocker, thus decreasing dysfunction of nerve impulses. It was originally used for spinal cord injuries.

This is prepared in an oral tablet or capsule and is still experimental. It can only be purchased with a prescription filled at a compounding pharmacy. It was originally used only for spinal cord injuries. Dosage must be started gradually and built up as overdose can cause convulsions.

I have been using this for four years now and feel very positive about its benefits, including better coordination and an increase in heat tolerance.

Natural Approach has a special connotation assigned to it called complementary and alternative medicine (CAM). This approach is not one to be used during times of exacerbations but to be used during periods of remission. In my experience, alternative therapies, herbs, restricted diet, and supplements can control the disease to a great extent.

Make sure vitamin D levels are optimized and regularly tested. Balancing the Omega-6 to Omega-3 ratios is important. Elimination of most commercial milk and dairy products is highly effective. Amino Ethanol Phosphate, bound with 10 percent calcium (Calcium AEP), can be helpful. Electromagnetic stimulation of the pineal gland can help, but it is expensive and must be used long term. Alpha lipoic acid decreases the phagocytosis of the myelin by macrophages. Progesterone promotes the formation of new myelin sheath.

Most drugs the doctors prescribe treat the symptoms, not the cause. One drug leads to having to take another and snowballs. A survey on nutrition done by MSWatch® with 4,468 people showed the following results: 40 percent felt diet was important, 38 percent felt their diet was well balanced, 33 percent chose diet to improve overall health, 68 percent did not discuss nutrition with their doctors. Seventy percent took vitamin supplements, 55 percent did not take mineral supplements, 74 percent did not take herbal supplements, 33 percent chose supplements to improve overall health, 43 percent have discussed supplements with their doctor, and 19 percent found information on supplements from books and magazines.

Therapeutic Goals

This list is something MS patients should strive for.
- Alleviate existing symptoms
- Detoxify with either a temporary fast or juice diet and eliminate food additives, preservatives, refined carbohydrates and saturated fats

- Eat a well-balanced diet that eliminates or reduces animal proteins, refined carbohydrates, stimulants, and all processed food and drinks while emphasizing fresh fruits, vegetables, and grains
- Exercise daily
- Have a positive mental attitude and reduce stress
- Keep the progress of the disease in check
- Reduce the number of episodes
- Stop the episode (if possible)
- Supplement with vitamins A, C, D, E, and B complex, the minerals magnesium, selenium, thymus extract, and zinc, and the enzymes amylase, bromelain, chymotrypsin, lipase, pancreatin, papain, and trypsin
- Discuss any medical condition concerns about MS with your qualified health care provider

Beneficial Supplements

Here is a list of supplements and dosage that my research found could be beneficial. Be sure to check with your health care provider about your personal dosage if you have any questions.

- Bilberry (50mg)
- Calcium orotate with 100 mg magnesium (0.5 g 3t/day)
- Cod liver oil (2 grams-1 tablespoon/day)
- DHEA (25 mg 2t/day)
- Evening primrose oil (2 tabs 3t/day)
- Flaxseed oil (10 grams)
- Ginkgo biloba (40-80mg 3t/day)
- Grape Seed Extract (50 mg)
- Lecithin (2 tabs 3t/day)
- Lipoic acid (100mg 2t/day)
- Magnesium (500mg)
- Multiple mineral combo supplements (as directed on container)
- Octacosanol (8000 mcg 2t/day)
- Olive leaf extract (1 tab 2t/day)
- Omega-3 (1t/day)
- Pancreatin (300-700mg 3t/day)
- Pregnanolone (10 mg 2t/day)
- Pycnogenol (100mg)

- Selenium (200-400 mcg/day)
- Vitamin A (5000 IU)
- Vitamin B3 – Niacinamide (500 mg/day)
- Vitamin B5 – Pantothinic acid (500 mg/day)
- Vitamin B6 (200 mg/day)
- Vitamin B12 (600 mcg/day minimum)
- Vitamin C (2000-6000mg/day)
- Vitamin D (1000-4000 IU/day)
- Vitamin E (400 IU 3t/day)
- Zinc (25mg)

Recommended Diet Change

Minerals such as zinc and selenium strengthen the immune system and help ward off viral infections. Occasional use of the herbs goldenseal, echinacea, and vitamin C are beneficial in assisting to fight off infections and the common cold. They should not be taken for periods longer than seven days without a break of at least five days. Goldenseal may be allergenic to some people.

Studies have shown that two chemicals, anthocyanocides and proanthocyanocides, strengthen the BBB. These chemicals are found in blueberries, cherries, black berries, grapes, and the bark and needles of certain pine trees. These chemicals can be derived from encapsulated herb supplements marketed as bilberry, grape seed extract, and pycnogenol. These are very powerful anti-oxidants.

Please read the chapters on food and nutrition in this guide for more information on diet.

Suggestions for Coping

Don't be embarrassed to ask for help. You will find most people are very willing to offer a hand, especially if you are polite and gracious. Do not be stubborn and let pride cloud your judgment. Some tasks that were taken for granted prior to MS are simply too difficult and could cause you harm.

If you are a parent, ask your children to help out of love and respect, not because they have to.

Look into rescheduling if you do not feel up to doing something. Slow down and be more careful; adjust your activities allowing more time to rest. Let someone else do tasks for you when possible. Realize your limits and let go of things you used to do that are too difficult.

When you are besieged with flares or full-blown exacerbations, get treatment to prevent further damage that you cannot rebuild. Flu shots are not dangerous for patients with MS but the flu can be.

CHAPTER 2
Author's Medical and MS History

This chapter discusses my own personal experience with treatments regarding multiple sclerosis. It also relates my other illnesses, fevers, and regular medical complications.

A Brief History of My MS and Medical Chronology

1938-1956: My childhood medical history was fairly normal in terms of diseases and medical problems. It included an adenoidectomy, an appendectomy, chickenpox, measles, and a tonsillectomy. A high intake of sweets caused cavities and the necessity for many fillings in my teeth at a time when mercury amalgam fillings were the normal procedure used by dentists. Mercury poisoning could have been one of the contributing causes of my future MS. During these years I required stitches twice to close wounds: the first from falling on an ice skate where the blade cut my nose, and the other from a cut to my nose from a hair dryer pipe. In high school, I cracked an anklebone playing football and chipped a bone in my thumb playing basketball.

1960: I was married the summer after I turned twenty-one. While practicing slow-pitch softball, I was hit in the back with a ball thrown in from the outfield. My family doctor said a pinched nerve could be what was causing the occasional tingling in my left hand and some balance problems.

1961: In January, I was laid off from work. In the spring I began misjudging fly balls and occasionally—inexplicably—I had blurred vision, temporary weakness, and at times my balance was off. My doctor, concerned about my well-being, recommended a well-known neurosurgeon. The neurosurgeon hospitalized me in May to run a series of tests. After two weeks with no positive diagnosis, I was released from the hospital with the diagnosis that I was suffering from Transverse Myelitis (spinal-cord inflammation). I then began treatment with a chiropractor: working on my spine, neck, leg flexibility, balance, and muscle tone.

1962: In December, I was hospitalized again; and, once again, there was no conclusive diagnosis. I continued treatments with a chiropractor.

1963: The chiropractor recommended I see an eye doctor. After a four-hour exam, he thought I had MS, but did not want to be the only one making the diagnosis. I called the neurologist. In June, I was hospitalized in order to undergo a spinal tap and the diagnosis of MS was confirmed. Treatment included cortisone injections, and after two days, I was back to what I felt was my normal self. I did remain in the hospital for the tapering off period.

1964: In October, noticing more balance problems, my neurologist started me on 4 mg of medrol; I improved temporarily. My doctor's exam showed changes to the discs in my eyes, so in November I was again hospitalized for nine days and given shots of ACTH.

1965: The next attack was in September, and I was hospitalized and once again given injections of ACTH.

1966: In March, I started having temporarily blurred vision and muscle weakness again, so I asked my doctor if I could give myself shots instead of going into the hospital. He gave me a prescription for 80 units of ACTH to be taken every twelve hours for five days. I had to repeat the ACTH treatment again in August and December. My doctor and I worked on that schedule for the next twenty-four years until the doctor retired. Stress, caused in part by marital discord, played a role at this time.

1967: I required shots of ACTH again in May and December of 40 units each time.

1968: I filed for divorce early in January. It was final in September.

1969: In March, I did 60 units of ACTH.

1970: In June, I went to Sweden for a job assignment and took the prescription with me. In September I did another ACTH treatment.

1971: In January, I returned to Sweden, under contract for three more months. In September I repeated ACTH again.

1974: I went back to Sweden for the third time on a job assignment. My neurologist gave me the following letter in case I might experience an exacerbation while I was away:

To Whom It May Concern:

   Mr. Charles Tiffany has a mild case of Multiple Sclerosis. In case of a significant exacerbation, he should be treated with ACTH gel 60 to 80 units every twelve hours (IM) for a course of ten to fourteen days. He should also during treatment be on a low salt diet and take a potassium supplement by mouth.

   Very truly yours,

   Richard A. Taylor, M.D.

1976: I had a few minor flare-ups, but no ACTH treatment again until October.

1977: I married an English lady I met on a bus tour in Scotland in the fall of 1975.

1982: In January, I had a bilateral hernia operation.

1983: In January, I had another bilateral inguinal hernia operation because the first one failed.

1984: My next requirement for ACTH was in August.
I also went to a local clinic for a swelling in my left elbow and shoulder and I was treated with a shot and a prescription.

1987: In August, I needed 40 units of ACTH again. I also went to the clinic with a sore throat. I received a shot and a prescription.

1988: In October, I went to the clinic and had my thyroid and cholesterol levels checked. I also had a urine test.

1989: In March, I went to the clinic with a sore throat and head congestion. After an x-ray of my sinuses, I was treated with a shot and a prescription. In September, I had a random glucose cholesterol test. Also in September, I had a lower GI (gastrointestinal series of x-rays), with a barium enema as a check for diverticula, but the doctors found none.

1990: In March, I went to the clinic with another sore throat, and was treated again with a shot and a prescription.
In July, I needed ACTH again with a dosage of 40 units. Prior to July, my MS was manageable. I still golfed and bowled until that time.

1991: In July, because of back pain, I had a cervical spine x-ray.

1992: During my next exacerbation I was under a new doctor's care because of my previous neurologist's retirement. I was admitted to the hospital in July for acute cholecystitis (gallbladder inflammation) and the exacerbation, yet no cholelithiasis or cholecystitis was found. Instead, the diagnosis was spastic paraparesis (viral infection of the spinal cord) and ataxia (coordination problems) with a urinary tract infection. While in the hospital I had a cholecystotomy (gall bladder removal) and was treated for a urinary tract infection. After treatment, I had to walk with a cane, as balance had become a major concern, along with incontinence.
This was my first exacerbation under this new doctor's care, and his treatment was with solumedrol IVs. I did not recover as I had in all my past treatments. I wonder why the ACTH treatments that in the past had worked so well fell out of favor.

1993: In December, I had a blood and biochemistry test profile (a test for general health), and my prostate was checked at the clinic.

1994: I was admitted to the hospital in May with a MS exacerbation and was released after a seven-day treatment with solumedrol IV and oral prednisone. I also had a urine test. An ankle-foot-orthotic (AFO) was not used yet, but I had some foot drop, a condition where you cannot voluntarily keep your ankle flexed while walking.

1995:   In August, I began treatment of physical therapy in order to try to help restore some of the muscle control that had been impaired by the effects of MS. In September, I was admitted to the hospital ER with chest pains and a possible blockage. I was given six days of EKG's (electrocardiogram image tests of electrical recordings of the heart). They wanted to operate, but I felt I needed a second opinion, so I was released. In October, I was re-admitted to hospital again with chest pains. The diagnosis was coronary artery disease and unstable angina. I had another EKG, cardiac catheterization, and a transluminal angioplasty of right hand coronary artery. I was given aspirin, heparin, IV nitroglycerin and beta-adrenergic blockers, Ecotrin®, Toprol-XL™ 100 mg, Nitro-Bid 6.5 mg t.i.d., nitrostat, and Lopressor™ 50 mg. Also in October I went to the heart clinic for a check-up, and I had another EKG.

1996:   In May, I started an outpatient three-treatment laser surgery of a basal cell carcinoma. The spot was healed after the final treatment.
In July, I had another flare-up; this time, I did seven days of outpatient treatment of solumedrol. This amounted to going to the hospital for a three-hour IV for a seven-day treatment, and was followed by twenty-one days of decreasing doses of medrol. After this treatment, I returned somewhat to my status prior to July.
In October, I was admitted to the hospital ER because I awoke from a nap at 2 P.M. with a 101.8°F temperature, and could not move. The EMS ambulance transported me to the hospital.
In November, I had an upper GI and Barium Esophagoscope (an x-ray examination of the esophagus) as a check for a hiatial hernia.
In December, I went to the clinic for a heart stress echo test.

1997:   In February, I went to the clinic for treatment of a sinus infection. I went to the heart clinic for an EKG and follow-up with the cardiologist. I had two sinus infections and took amoxicillian to clear up the infections.
In October, I repeated outpatient treatment for my MS.

1998:   In March, I went to the clinic with another sore throat and sinus infection. Also in March, I was checked for a hernia because of a pain in my pelvic area. In April, cysts and moles were removed from my back and tested.

In August, I received treatment again for a sore throat and sinus infection. On November 14, I went to the clinic and received treatment for a sore throat and sinus infection. I was given a shot of antibiotics and a prescription. On November 21, I went back to the clinic and I was given another shot and new prescription for an experimental drug. On November 28 and then again on December 12, still not better, I was given yet another shot and a new prescription. On December 19, I was given another shot and had an x-ray taken of my stomach. On December 20, my coordination was terrible; I had a fever and was hospitalized. I was given a sinus CT (computed tomography), abdomen/pelvis CT, blood test, another x-ray of my stomach. The doctors decided I had some kind of infection with a possible penicillin allergy. The antibiotic therapy was changed to an IV of zithromax from vancomycin. The combination of taking dilantin and antibiotics from the doctor was the probable cause of my severe macular papillary rash (Red Man syndrome). It turned out to be a urinary tract infection. Pain across the lower area of my stomach was still unexplained. On December 21, I had a cat-scan and laparoscopy (exploratory surgery for possible appendix problems). The doctors found nothing wrong except an allergy to sulfonamides. A catheter was installed with a Foley leg bag (to catch the urine). I had to wear the Foley bag and catheter for two weeks. They found a small cyst on my kidney, but I was told not to worry about it. Once again, a urinary tract infection was the problem. I was released from the hospital on January 2, 1999. I was given a prescription for Detrol® LA for overactive bladder, hydroxyzine (an antihistamine), zithromax for rash, and beconaise for my nose.

1999: In January, I returned to the urologist to have the catheter removed and I tried to urinate, but with no luck. They taught me how to self-cathorize and I was given a prescription for triamcinolone to treat the fungus found in my urine. I also was given a prescription for macrobid to treat the urinary tract infection, and flomax to treat the prostate.
In March, I started using beconaise regularly to help prevent sinus problems. After March 13, I no longer had to use the catheter.
In May, I had a minor flare-up of shingles for which I received a 15 cc-shot of Celestone and a prescription.

In October, I had a Social Security Disability (SSDI) exam. Also in October, I had my first flu shot. Along with that I had a urine test and a pneumonia shot. In late October, I went to the Imaging Center for an ultra sound and a sonography of my kidneys. I started bactrim and finished the cycle in November. On November 3, I needed help dressing and I was taken to the hospital after having a fever during the night. I was started on zithromax. I had a sinus CT, a urine test, and a blood test. A urinary tract infection was found to be the cause for the fever. Late in November I went back for a urine test.

2001:   In March, I had another urine test. I started Mycelex® for a fungus yeast coating on my tongue along with Nystatin. Mycelex was discontinued at my doctor's request. I also did an outpatient treatment for my MS exacerbation.

In May, I started Avonex®. I had mixed feelings about using Avonex because of the possible side effects, but I agreed to give it a try. My hope was if I could go two years without an exacerbation by taking the shots, maybe I could go four years. If side effects or post-treatment discomfort became unbearable, I had agreed to stop taking the shots.

There were some minor side effects after first shot and a general feeling of depression and lethargy the rest of the week. St. Johns Wort (a herb for depression), Tylenol® and rest seemed to combat symptoms. In the fifth week of treatment I experienced a strange feeling: I had thoughts of suicide. This had popped up the week before for a brief instant; I had not given it much thought. But this time the thought lingered and I even began to think about how I might do it. I mentioned this to some people on the "MSWatch®" chat page and they insisted I call my doctor. I called the Avonex help desk and talked to a nurse who also said for me to call my doctor. The doctor returned my call and asked me to come into his office. This was on a Thursday. I wanted to stop the Avonex shots and see if that was the cause. He was not too keen on that and wanted to hospitalize me, but he agreed to let me stop the shots and call him Monday morning. This decision was agreeable with me. Maybe the problem was mental, because on Friday I went to the drug store, bank, physical therapy, and got gas for my van. It is possible that the relief of not taking the shots was at the bottom of my problems. This was my only experience with taking Avonex or any of the recommended treatments for extending remissions.

In July, a basal cell carcinoma was removed from my back in the shoulder area and it tested positive for cancer. In October, I had a blood test. In December, I had an allergy test that showed a slight notice of dog fluff.

2002:   In January, I started having more problems with impaired balance and falling. In February, my coordination was terrible and I had trouble dealing with stairs and incontinence. In March, I needed help with dressing and mobility. My wife stayed home from work and took me to my doctor. I was sent directly to the hospital to start a five-day outpatient treatment of solumedrol. Three days after the treatment, I was still having problems. The neurologist put me in the hospital for the seven-day treatment in order to watch my progress. I suffered repeated temperature spikes. I was released in stable condition, but still having temperature spikes. Home care visits provided a nurse and therapist.

I checked with the pharmacist on the ingredients of the 4-AP (4-aminopyridine) that I had been taking for so long. At the beginning of the year I had upped my dosage to 4t/day rather than 3 t/day. Although this was about the same time my temperature started to spike, I had not related this to my problems since it was not on a daily basis. The pharmacist said the 4-AP was mixed with lactose. I was lactose intolerant and apparently my body was fighting the drug, causing the spikes. He suggested taking Lactaid® along with the 4-AP, and this worked great.

I still visited the neurologist for regular check-ups.

Present MS Status

For the past four years, I have been getting a shot of 40 units of depomedrol whenever I feel a minor flare-up. That seems to quiet the flare quickly. I can go to the local medical clinic and get a shot of depomedrol and a B12 shot. I also take Tylenol if there is any kind of rise in body temperature because body heat causes my legs to go weak.

I have some tingling and weakness that is more pronounced on my left side. My mobility is compromised since my coordination is impaired. I have to use a four-post walker without wheels to get around the house and for short trips. I use a wheelchair for longer trips. When I go out on my own, I use my walker for short distances and to get from the driver's seat to the rear hatch on my van where there is an electric lift for removal of my electric wheelchair. I still drive with the standard controls and an automatic transmission. My right ankle is still flexible and strong enough to switch from the gas pedal to the brake without having to lift my leg.

I wear an AFO on my left leg all the time to aid foot drop. I have a "K" brace that keeps my right knee from hyper-extending. I usually wear the "K" brace in the mornings around the house.

When traveling on a plane, I wear a pull-up type of brief for peace of mind. I can manage the aisle by holding onto the seat backs as I travel to the bathroom. I don't eat or drink anything prior to travel because bowel incontinence can be a problem. Furthermore, my left leg collapses once in a while, so I have to be aware of that possibility.

There is a small stall shower in my bathroom, adjacent to the main bedroom, which has a grab bar, shower seat, and heavy-duty doors. I stand to shower and then sit to do my legs and feet. The water has to be lukewarm or the heat bothers my leg coordination.

The numbness in my arms, fingers, hands, and feet is noticeably better than what it was a year ago. I carry a bedpan and urinal in the car and have had to use them occasionally. I have not had to lie down in the afternoons now for well over two years, and have not had a cold or sinus condition. I go to physical therapy twice a week or exercise on my own.

I cannot provide any insight into drugs for balance, depression, muscle weakness, pain, or other MS related symptoms, since I have not experienced these symptoms to a severity that necessitates their use.

Present Medical Status

My present health is quite good except for having MS. My weight of 132 pounds at my height of 5'6" is good and my blood pressure is normally 120/80. The results of my blood test on April 5, 2002, were: cholesterol 196<200, triglycerides 153<200, LDL 80<130, HDL 85>34. My normal body temperature is 97.8°F. At temperatures even slightly above this, I notice problems, so care must be taken. This seems quite common for PWMS.

My MS Treatment Philosophy

Multiple sclerosis doesn't just happen to someone overnight: it takes years to develop the symptoms that lead to a diagnosis. A trusted health practitioner has told me that the rate of healing is one month for every year of a pathogen. It takes over fourteen years and $500 million for an experimental drug to get from the laboratory to the patient. If researchers find a vaccine or some other cure, it may be too late for a person with MS to revert back to the way he or she was.

Those with MS should look for ways to enhance their quality of life. My philosophy is to focus on improvement. It will take time. In my opinion, choosing to do nothing at all is a greater risk than acting on behalf of your own health and overall well being.

Self-improvement is a process that will take time to implement, and the steps involved are not easy. I believe MS requires a lifestyle change. Think of it as sliding downhill: if you continue on with what you are doing, it follows that you will continue to go downhill. It is important to keep a positive outlook on the possibilities for enhanced health.

CHAPTER 3
Author's Alternative Treatment History

This chapter contains information related to the time in my life that I started looking into alternative ways to improve my overall health. I am not recommending that you try these alternative treatments, I am only recounting what I have tried.

1990: A co-worker friend mentioned it might be beneficial for me to see her reflexologist. This was the beginning of my foray into alternative treatment supplements. After taking the products she suggested, I gradually started to feel better and seemed to be healthier. Both my wife and my mother noticed the improvement, so they joined me going to see the reflexologist. The reflexologist did iridology (examination of the iris as a primary diagnostic aid) and took pictures of my eyes and explained some of the problems she saw. To reduce costs, I enrolled in two of the multi-level marketing (MLM) companies for the products she recommended: Sunrider and Nature's Sunshine. Though we benefited from the Sunrider products, we decided to stop taking them because of price hikes. We still use the products and membership from Nature's Sunshine. The three of us went to the reflexologist monthly, but because of travel distance and cost, we tapered off until we stopped going all together.

1995: Prior to my angioplasty in September of 1995, I had received twelve treatments of chelation (an IV of EDTA—further explained in Chapter 10) to rid my body of metal toxicity. It is surprising this did not prevent the chest pains I had in September. After the angioplasty, I had chelation treatments weekly for the next six months, then on a twice-monthly basis for a year, and now on a once-monthly basis. Over the years, I have had more than one hundred chelation treatments.
After going to a house party demonstration for magnetic therapy (small magnet inserts that fit into your shoes) and meeting an osteopathic doctor (DO), my wife and I bought a pair to try. I experienced a very slight, temporary boost in energy.
I went to the clinic where the DO worked, and chose to see another

doctor. The doctor informed me that mercury was still causing problems even after I'd had my fillings removed. He suggested ten injections of sodium dimercaptopropanesulfonate (DMPS) and hair analysis, before and after, to determine the results. The DMPS was successful in removing half the mercury that had appeared in the hair analysis. The doctor recommended I continue the chelation treatments after the DMPS. I received chelation treatments at the clinic. If I was feeling under the weather, I would get an immune boost IV (concentrated vitamins and minerals). I have had around twenty of these treatments over an eight-year period.

The clinic was a pleasure to visit. Everyone was very friendly and there were two rooms of people getting treated with chelation, immune boosts, or other alternative treatments, which provided lots of conversation. One of the nurses was bubbly and I asked to what she attributed that. She said she drank a glass of ozonated water three times a day. The ozone generator puts oxygen into the water. I purchased one and still use it but not on a regular basis.

In November, I had a Darkfield blood test (a drop of blood placed under a microscope) that prompted the first of five treatments of photoluminescence (passing blood under an ultraviolet light—further explained in Chapter 8). Another Darkfield test, after the five treatments, showed an increase in the quality of my blood.

1997:   In January, I saw a nutritionist who did kinesiology (the science of using muscle testing). He charged $75 an hour and tried acupuncture and supplements from another MLM company. He also recommended a colon cleanse using the Clean-Me-Out Program. I bought and read the book *Cleanse & Purify Thyself* by Dr. Richard Anderson, N.D., N.M.D. It was a method of self-healing through intestinal cleansing and digestive rejuvenation. I bought the supplies from the nutritionist and started the program. The first three weeks I could eat only two meals a day of fruits and vegetables, along with the supplements and a drink mixture from the kit. I could drink all the purified water I wanted. The fourth week only one meal a day was allowed, again fruits and vegetables. During the fifth week no food was allowed, only the supplements and the mixture. Enemas had to be done twice a day, morning and evening, for all five weeks. If I did not do this, the toxins in my body made me feel terrible. I know this sounds like a lot of hassle and effort, but the results were amazing. After the first couple of days, my energy skyrocketed and weight loss was noticeable. I lost six pounds the first week and nineteen pounds overall. I lost two inches around my waist and felt great. My only problem was halfway through the fifth week when I had to start eating food because I was getting weak.

In April, I started the first of a hundred treatments of "KI." This is a Japanese form of energy treatment in which the practitioner transfers energy from his or her body to the recipient's body. This may sound strange, but I saw the practitioner move people from six feet away, raise a person's head, and make a person roll over without touching the person. All of this seems a little strange and hard to believe, but after viewing many demonstrations with my own eyes, I can say that it can happen. Treatments were three times a week for a five to eight minute session. This gave some temporary relief from symptoms, but it did not last.

2000: I read information about the procarin patch. One of my alternative care doctors asked me if I would like to give it a try. I noticed slight improvements for the first six weeks, then nothing, so I stopped the treatments after three months.

In the fall, I had two more treatments of photoluminescence with two more in early 2001. I felt no immediate benefits other than continued good health.

My first treatment of hydrogen peroxide (an IV of diluted hydrogen peroxide that converts to oxygen inside the body—further explained in Chapter 9) was in December of 1998; other than a short boost in energy, my MS symptoms did not change, so I stopped these treatments. After reading a book on the benefits of hydrogen peroxide and starting research for this book, I decided to once again give it a try. I hoped to get rid of a long-time yeast infection. I used this treatment in combination with the drug Nystatin to try to clear up the yeast infection. It helped, but without sticking to a yeast free diet, the yeast infection survived.

In September, I started using a zapper (a small battery operated frequency device—further explained in Chapter 11), along with a new diet regime. Zapping kills parasites that are living in the body. I felt I had more feeling in my hands and arms, better mobility, easier movement on stairs, coordination improvements, increased energy, and no further need for naps.

Positive results were noticed the second day. I still do the zapping, but not on a regular basis. (See the zapper log in the appendix for improvement details.)

I found the book *The Cure for all Diseases* by Hulda Clark to be interesting. Another book I found beneficial is *New Hope, Real Help for Those That Have Multiple Sclerosis* by John Pageler. Pageler gives advice about which supplements he recommends, what they are for, and the dosage. This book is now out of print. I have tried to incorporate some of Pageler's advice into this book.

Another alternative that has been very helpful to me is 4-Aminopyridine (4-AP). It is a potassium channel blocker that improves conduction of electrical impulses through nerves and was shown to improve clinical signs and symptoms in MS patients, such as ambulation, fatigue, and visual function. It has been found helpful with patients of longstanding disease and heat sensitivity. Still experimental, the prescription has to be filled by a compounding pharmacy, and it is imperative that the dosage be started gradually.

Effects of oral 4-AP normally last four to seven hours. Possible side effects are mild dizziness or tingling; however, a more serious side effect, convulsions, usually happens when doses are started too high or taken too close together. Test results showed two in twenty-three patients suffered a generalized epileptic seizure and one patient contracted hepatitis. The other twenty patients showed a favorable response. After a long continuation of use, stopping this medication may cause symptoms to return.

I took one 10 mg tablet a day for two weeks, then two tablets a day for the next two weeks, then three a day and I stayed there until early 2002, when I began taking four tablets a day at five-hour intervals, which is where I remain today. It noticeably helps my coordination. If I forget to take a tablet every five hours, my hand and leg coordination is definitely impaired. I have been taking 4-AP for over four years, and I feel very positive about its usefulness.

I have had one treatment of Reiki, a technique for improving health by balancing out energy systems. It is a holistic therapy that harmonizes body, mind and spirit, using non-polarized energy from the palms of the hands of the therapist. It was a good experience but benefits were temporary. Another treatment I have just started is quantum electro dynamics (QED), a holistic biofeedback therapy that uses a Quantum Xrroid Consciousness Interface (QXCI) machine. (This machine was further explained in Chapter 1.) Though only a few treatments have been completed, the physical benefits are already noticeable. I plan on continuing with the hope of getting better. (See the log sheets in the appendix for specific results.)

Alternatives Tried and Discarded

Bee venom injections did not work for me. I tried five injections the first time, ten the second time and fifteen the third time. The day after my last injections, I was unable to get out of bed on my own, so I decided to stop. The injections were given at different points along the side of my left leg and down my back. The injections were not uncomfortable because Novocain was rubbed on the injection spot. Some PWMS benefit from this treatment.

Other alternatives I have tried are products sold by the following list of companies: Amway, Body Wise, Cell-Tech, Enrich, Mannatech, Morinda, Sun Chlorella, and Sunrider.

Alternative Supplements

A list of the supplements I am presently taking follows. This list is revised occasionally:

- Psyllium hulls combo (1 tsp.) for fiber and bowels
- Liquid chlorophyll (1/2 oz.) for bursitis in arm and general well-being
- Liquid aminos (1/2 oz.) for energy and amino supplementation
- Acidolphus (4) for intestinal purposes
- E-tea (4) for cancer prevention
- Vitamin E (3 @ 400 IU) for heart
- Vitamin C (2 @ 1000 mg Super Gram II) for immune system
- Supersupplemental (1) for vitamins and well-being
- Saw Palmetto (2) for prostate
- HP Garlic (1) for heart and circulation

- Vitamin D (2 @ 400 IU) for general health and MS
- Calcium + Vitamin D + Magnesium (3) for bones and MS
- Potassium (1) for general health and it is needed with calcium
- Magnesium (3 @ 250 mg) for muscle control
- Lecithin (3) for general health
- CoQ10 (1 @ 100 mg) for heart
- Pancreatin (3) for general health and MS
- Evening primrose (3) for digestion and MS
- Octocosanal (2 @ 2000 mcg) for myelin build
- Omega-3 (2) for general health
- Valerian Root (2) for nerves
- Vitamin B Complex (2) for nervous system
- Vitamin B12 (4) for energy
- DHEA (2 @ 25 mg) for hormones
- Pregnanolone (2 @ 30 mg) for myelin strengthening
- Olive Leaf Extract (1) for yeast
- Lipoic acid (1) for general health

My normal prescription drug supplementation is as follows:
- Flomax 0.4 mg (2) for urinary and kidney
- 4-Aminopyridine (4 @ 10 mg) for MS coordination and heat sensitivity
- Alprazolam (generic for Xanax) (0.25 mg) as needed for nerves

Present Alternative Treatment Status

Even with many physical compromises, I have a general feeling of well-being. I attribute this to alternative treatments that I have researched and undertaken on my own. I have been on herbal and supplemental programs since 1990. I still maintain my normal medical treatments for exacerbations.

Lately I try to arrange a treatment of hydrogen peroxide once a month. This gives a slight boost to my energy. It also seems to help in the prevention of acquiring colds or other infections. My overall coordination has been better. For years I have been zapping and getting one chelation treatment a month. I also take 4-AP. This greatly helps coordination, muscle impulses, and heat sensitivity. I also have been exercising regularly.

I am presently looking into the stem cell therapy. There may be the possibility of this helping to regain some of my physical losses. It is still in the research stages and much is not known, as yet.

CHAPTER 4
FOOD

This chapter contains information on improving the quality of the food you consume. The Zone Diet mentioned in this chapter is a more balanced way to eat. There are many diets on the market to help you lose weight if that is what you are interested in.

What You Eat

Do you eat what you like, or do you eat what you should to be healthy? Most of us probably fall into the first category. When we were young, our mothers tried to make sure we ate balanced meals. We were told to finish our meat and vegetables before we could have dessert. Now that we are adults, the scenario is different. We control what, when, and how we eat.

The majority of us are a little overweight. We might feel that a little splurge now and then doesn't hurt us. The problem is, in some cases, the splurges are not just a rarity, they're a habit. America is the most prosperous country in the world, and our waistlines show it.

Here is a formula to test if you should lose weight:

Your weight in pounds (135) x 0.45 = X
Your height in inches (66) x 0.025 = Y
Square Y (Y x Y) = Y2
Divide X by Y2 (X/Y2) = Z

Z should fall between nineteen and twenty-five. If your number is over twenty-five, you should lose weight. For the numbers above, Z works out to be 60.75 / 2.7225 = 22.31.

Positive Steps to Improve Health

If you want to improve your health, you may have to change. You must take the responsibility for your health; no one else is going to plot out a roadmap for you. If you start to make changes to improve your heath and slip, don't panic or give up, just start over.

If you take care of your body, it will take care of you. The partnership with your body is a lot like a marriage: it requires a great amount of care and attention. The body is very forgiving and has remarkable rejuvenation powers. Roughly six out of ten deaths in the United States are related to diet. Dieting and calorie counting generally do not last or bring about the desired results. If we eat the correct amount of proteins, carbohydrates, and fat, we'll experience many benefits: better sleep and moods, less fatigue, sickness, cravings, stress, irritability, more energy, and our weight will balance.

There are a couple of sayings: "diet cures what diet causes" and "you wear tomorrow what you eat today," which mean that if you start eating right, your health and your image will gradually improve. It does not happen instantly, but it will happen.

Some basics for improving your health are: drink lots of water and eliminate alcohol, chocolate, coffee, milk, sugar, tea (with caffeine), and all white flour products from your diet, or at least cut down. Coffee gives you an instant lift, so what's wrong with it? Caffeine depletes energy and is a great cause of stress. Decaffeinated is even more caustic then regular coffee because dangerous chemicals are used to remove the caffeine. Caffeine has detrimental effects on the heart such as: raising blood pressure, increasing the heart rate, and contributing to heart disease. It causes a temporary surge in blood sugar, increases the secretion of hydrochloric acid, and depletes calcium from the body. Extended caffeine consumption, over time, leads to adrenal exhaustion and the depletion of B-vitamins, especially B-5, which supports adrenal health. Caffeine dehydrates the body and leads to premature aging. It is an addictive drug that works like amphetamines—cocaine and heroin, for example—to stimulate the brain.

Fat and sugar, in slightly elevated proportions, cause problems for the heart because they raise cholesterol. Hydrogenated oils, trans-fatty acids, white rice, and white flour should also be avoided. Refined white sugar and enriched white flour strip our bodies of B-complex vitamins. Research studies show hydrogenated oils and trans-fatty acids cause non-insulin dependent Type II diabetes. White rice has had the bran layer stripped during the milling process. This bran layer contains vital nutritional elements. White flour is a simple carbohydrate that has been through a bleaching process and stripped of many natural vitamins.

A low-fat diet can be very helpful to people with lupus, multiple sclerosis, rheumatoid arthritis, and scleroderma. A study of multiple sclerosis patients showed a marked decrease in function for those individuals who chose not to remain on the low-fat diet.

Learn the basics of food assimilation. Eat fruits first at a meal, vegetables and carbohydrates next, and get protein from good sources. (Later in this chapter, I will give examples of good fats, proteins, and carbs.) If you must eat meat, do so last. Chew your food well, as digestion starts in the mouth, and do not drink liquids with your meal as they dilute the enzymes needed for digestion. Start substituting vegetarian recipes on a regular basis, and exercise!

Additional Steps for Improving Health

If you want to go one step further, do not eat a heavy meal upon rising or before going to bed. Eat only when you are hungry and then do not overeat. Do not eat saturated fats. Avoid highly processed and precooked foods. Steam, broil, or bake your food, and try to avoid fried foods. Cleanse your system occasionally by fasting with pure, fresh juices. Avoid alcohol, caffeine, cigarettes, drugs, and stress. Get plenty of fresh air and sunshine.

Some Additional Advice to Help Your Body

- Check out the labels in your cupboards. Products with aluminum, antibacterial properties, canola oil, fluoride, hydrogenated oils, soybean oil, mineral oil, or petroleum products will add toxic material to your body.
- Consider juicing raw fruits and vegetables for quick meals or snacks.
- Slow down activities to remove stress and get adequate rest.
- Add three to five tablespoons of dry ground ginger to your bath and soak for twenty minutes. This, along with dry skin brushing, will help rid toxins from your skin. Use a Ph-balanced soap. Dry skin brushing is a technique of using a natural bristle brush just prior to a shower or bath, prompting the body to release its toxic deposits and remove dry skin.
- Add Braggs liquid aminos to your diet; it is a healthy liquid soybean condiment that contains sixteen amino acids and is a powerful additive in the fight against arteriosclerosis and other degenerative diseases. Braggs has fat-burning action and helps restore function to blood vessel walls. It can also help reduce the risk of potential angina for coronary patients. It can be used on salads or added to a glass of water or juice.
- Another product I like is liquid chlorophyll. It contains life-giving nutrients that help control and regulate calcium levels. It also serves to lubricate the ileocecal valve (the valve between the large and small intestine) and contains minerals to

help build new cells. It is a great natural healer: it helps purify the liver, keep the colon healthy, regulate the bowels, and deter the development of toxic bacteria. The percentage of disease caused by constipation and colon toxicity is very high. It normally takes three to six months to rebuild the bowel and colon to adequate tone and elasticity. One ounce of liquid chlorophyll is equal to one cup of green tea. It too can be added to water.

- Romaine lettuce has more beta-carotene, foliate, and vitamin C than iceberg lettuce.
- Pink grapefruit has more beta-carotene than white grapefruit.
- Vegetables lose much of their mineral content when boiled versus steamed.
- Low-sodium V8 juice is a good alternative to soda pop and each glass equals a full serving of vegetables. Drink a 6-ounce can of low-sodium tomato juice, vegetable juice, or V8 as a pick-me-up.
- Add frozen carrot slices, peas, or string beans to soups heated in a microwave.
- Add more vegetables to your recipes than called for in the directions.
- Add chopped apples, diced mango, grape halves, or pineapple cubes to your chicken salad.
- Add a lot of chopped celery, jicama or onions to your tuna salad.
- Try grapefruit in the morning before cereal.
- Replace candy when craved with fruits like cherries, cranberries, papayas, or raisins.

I do not profess to know exactly what you should eat, but I do know that any time spent reading and practicing good food management will benefit you greatly. A couple of books I found helpful are *The Zone* by Barry Sears, Ph.D. with Bill Lawren; *Zone Perfect Meals in Minutes* by Barry Sears, Ph.D.; *Adkins for Life* by Robert C. Adkins, M.D.; and *The Multiple Sclerosis Diet Book* by Roy Laver Swank, M.D., Ph.D. and Barbara Brewer Dugan.

What we eat is as important as how and when. You are better off eating less and eating right.

Eating meals at approximately the same time each day helps the body use the food to gain the best results. Try to eat every four to six hours. Eating a lot of food at one meal then missing a meal is harmful; eating four small meals is preferable to two big ones. Snacking between meals is not bad as long as it is done in moderation, and once again, the protein/carbohydrates/fat (PCF) is correct. Some fast food items are tolerable if put into the correct ratio of PCF. In the Zone diet these numbers are 30 percent each of fat and protein with carbohydrates being 40 percent.

Foods that are rich in protein are chicken, crab, egg whites, fish, lean beef or ham, lobster, low-fat cottage cheese, soybean powder, tofu, tuna, and turkey.

Foods that are rich in nutritious carbohydrates are beans (black, kidney, navy, pinto, and soy), bread (pita or whole grain), oats and oatmeal, rice (brown or wild), peas, yams, and yogurt (low or non-fat).

Carbohydrates are processed by enzymes in your gastrointestinal tract into small particles that are absorbed in your bloodstream. This process results in a rise in blood glucose, and glucose is where your energy comes from. Some carbohydrates cause a fast rise and fall in glucose. Favorable carbohydrates have a low Glycemic Index.

Tests have been done to derive a Glycemic Index number for almost all foods. The Glycemic Index rates how fast carbohydrates break down into glucose and increase blood sugar levels. A lower number means the conversion is slower and energy is longer lasting. Larger numbers will give you a temporary high. Some examples of this Glycemic Index number are yams (73 & 51), beets (91 & 64), and cooked carrots (56 & 39). The first number is the overall Glycemic number in relation to all foods, and the second number relates to foods within that food group. A list of all foods can be found at www.mendosa.com. A fruit can have the same Glycemic Index number as a vegetable or bread.

The list of fruits and vegetables is wide open, so there are many choices. It is a good idea to wash your fruits and vegetables off in a mild solution of food-grade hydrogen peroxide and water before cooking or eating to clean any surface contamination they may have.

The amount of fat you eat should be based on your height and weight. Saturated fats should be kept to a minimum. Fat contains nine calories per gram. Protein contains only four calories per gram. Fat is the primary source of energy for your muscles.

Your body needs potassium. It helps balance sodium. Eating too much sodium (salt) can be a contributing factor in asthma, hypertension, kidney disease, stomach cancers, and ulcers. When the sodium intake is too high, the body excretes it through the urine, taking calcium with it, possibly causing osteoporosis. Excess salt has been linked to high blood pressure. A good ratio of sodium to potassium is one to four. You get natural potassium from fruits, nuts, vegetables, and whole grains. Follow guidelines to healthy eating and increase the healthy food you put in your body.

Remember, you are what you eat. Read the labels on products and know how to interpret what is in the package. If you can keep your calorie count down and your fat intake at a level that is considered normal, you will benefit greatly.

Factors That Cause Health Problems

In order to market certain foods, they have to be frozen, dried, or chemically treated to preserve them until they are cooked or readied for consumption. Most meat today is filled with additives, antibiotics, dyes, hormones, pesticides, tranquilizers, and other harmful substances. Farmers spray or treat their crops to enhance output and increase their financial gains. Money drives many of our processes, not health. A large percentage of processed food in our grocery stores has genetically engineered ingredients added. They include soy beans, potatoes, soft drinks, ketchup, potato chips, cookies, ice cream, and corn, just to mention a few.

Gene splicing is another form of genetically enhancing certain foods to grow faster or bigger. This biotechnology science is changing our food. Some plants have pesticides engineered into them that repel insects. Biotech foods in Europe and Japan have been causing outbreaks of protests. This biotech revolution has not been around long enough for us to know what the effect is going to be. Products do not have to be labeled as such for biotech processing.

Some foods contain high levels of acrylamide, a chemical found in some fried or processed foods. It is one of the possible causes of cancer when consumed in high doses.

Unhealthy Habits

Many foods are rich in fat and will cause your body harm if consumed on a regular basis. A formula to watch and use, when you are shopping and reading labels is to multiply the fats (number of grams) by nine, and divide that figure by the number of calories in the product. The resulting figure will be the percentage of calories from fat. The lower the number, the better the product is for you. Products high in saturated fat will cause your cholesterol level to rise and produce platelets in your blood that can be prerequisites to heart attacks and strokes.

Heart disease is the number one cause of death in the United States. Factors increasing the risk of heart disease are elevated homocysteine (a toxic amino acid that a simple blood test can check) and lipoprotein (a class of proteins that contain a lipid combined with a simple protein) with low antioxidant levels in the body.

Statins (cholesterol-lowering drugs) are very popular (Baycol, Lescol, Lipitor, Mevacor, Pravachol, and Zocor). Possible side effects of statin drugs include blurred vision, intestinal gas, liver damage, liver toxicity, muscle inflammation, myopathy, rash, and weakness. These drugs block the body's ability to produce essential CoQ10. Some people have even died from this. These products also deplete the body, by up to 40 percent, of CoQ10 which is essential for the heart and energy production in the body.

Cardiomyopathy (damage to the heart) is one of the primary causes of heart failure that can be caused by a deficiency in CoQ10. Natural supplementation of CoQ10, fiber, folic acid, vitamin B6, vitamin B12, vitamin C, and vitamin E help keep homocysteine levels in check. It is a good idea to have your alanine aminotransferase (ALT—an enzyme that becomes elevated with liver disease), cholesterol, glucose, high-density lipoprotein (HDL), low-density lipoprotein (LDL), triglycerides, and cholesterol/HDL ratios checked. ALT range should be between 0–53, cholesterol should be 200 or below, glucose range should be 65–125, HDL should be greater than 34, LDL should be below 130, triglycerides should be below 200 and the cholesterol/HDL ratio should be in the 4.0–6.7 range. Just as an added note of interest, the cholesterol number used to be 220, and it has since been lowered to 200.

Fluoride is a poison; although 50 percent of the fluoride we ingest is excreted, the other 50 percent remains stored, mainly in the bones. Skeletal fluorosis and hip fractures are a serious risk for persons that have ingested 10-20 mg of fluoride for ten to twenty years.

Sugar (white cane) and white flour are two of the worst things to put in your body. Sugar weakens your body's immune system, in turn weakening your resistance to viruses and bacteria. The average American eats about a hundred pounds of sugar a year. Sugar is found in bread, cereal, ketchup, peanut butter, and spaghetti sauce, just to note some common products. Other forms of sugar are dextran, dextrin, dextrose, fructose, galactose, honey, maltose, and lactose. Sugar increases adrenaline and the production of cholesterol and cordisone. Sugar has been so highly processed there is nothing good for you left in it. (See the appendix: Fifty-Six Reasons Sugar Ruins Your Health.)

Aspartame, Equal, and NutraSweet are substitutes, but still not good for you. Aspartame breaks down into methanol (alcohol) once in the body where it is further metabolized into formaldehyde. NutraSweet has methanol, an alcohol, as one of its ingredients. Two of the other ingredients are phenylalanine and aspartic acid.

Along these same lines are the harmful ingredients that are found in soft drinks. These include artificial color, flavoring, caffeine, phosphoric acid, and sugar. A healthy alternative for sugar is stevia, a sweet food from South America. It is much sweeter than sugar, a little goes a long way, and it is not harmful.

Red meats should not be ingested on a regular basis, as they are hard to digest. Fruits take half an hour to digest, vegetables take one hour, and meats take six to eight hours.

Cow's milk is another product that may be an active contributor to a multitude of diseases and disorders because of its high sugar content and allergenic proteins. Milk may contain an infectious agent, a toxic substance, or fats, which alter the nervous system. It can be a contributing factor in the cause of acne, anemia, atherosclerosis, bronchitis, cancer, cataracts, constipation, cramps, dental decay, diarrhea, ear infections, gastrointestinal bleeding, iron-deficiency, leukemia, multiple sclerosis, rheumatoid arthritis, and skin rashes.

It has always been known that milk contains vitamin D, but fortified, pasteurized, homogenized with vitamin D added may increase your risk of osteoporosis. The vitamin D in milk is D2 that is inferior to D3. A good source of vitamin D is a tablespoon of cod liver oil. It provides approximately 1350 IU of vitamin D. Other milk substitutes include soymilk and rice milk.

Tips for Health

Many parts of the body are taken for granted and sometimes neglected. Smoking causes damage to your lungs. Your thyroid and pituitary glands, though small, are very important and need help as you get older because their functionality decreases. Your liver and kidneys are very important, as they rid the body of wastes and toxins. Your colon is a long storage tube, and through its walls, your body is fed. It is like the pipe in advertisements for blocked drains. Once the walls of the colon are constricted by build up, the flow is interrupted. The walls cake up and become hard.

Your skin is also very important, as it is the largest waste disposal part of the body. When you sweat, toxins and other unwanted body products are excreted through the skin. The waste and elimination process greatly influences a large part of how you feel. If this system is not working properly, weakened organs and tissue begin showing symptoms such as: colitis, constipation, Crohn's disease, diarrhea, digestive disorders, diverticulitis, hemorrhoids, incontinence, irritable bowel syndrome, kidney malfunction, parasites, and varicose veins.

CHAPTER 5
NUTRITION

This chapter outlines basic nutrition and lists important vitamins and minerals. Almost all of the information in this chapter has been collected from articles, books, newsletters, publications, television, and the Internet.

Basic Nutrition

Taking care of your body is a lot like taking care of your car. Gas makes it run, oil must be changed. You check the fluids, keep air in the tires, wash it, and put on protective wax. Nutrition works the same for our bodies. We must maintain tuned-up vehicles or we will have breakdowns.

The Recommended Daily Allowance (RDA) published by the National Academy of Sciences is a guideline that serves as the basis for understanding what our bodies need to maintain a healthy life. The RDA is based on a two-thousand-calorie diet, and in general, these recommendations are on the low side for most individuals. These figures were published nearly fifty years ago, and under most circumstances, due to lifestyles today and nutritional intake, they need to be increased.

The "Suggested Need" column in the following chart is my own list compiled over four years of research. The following list is for adults. If you have questions, please confirm with a healthcare provider or nutritionist.

Nutrient	RDA	Suggested Need
Biotin	200 mcg	200-300 mcg
Bromelain	0	200 mg
Calcium	800 mg	1000-2000 mg
Chloride	1700 mg	2500 mg
Choline	150 mg	600 mg
Chromium	50 mcg	200 mcg
Copper	2 mg	3-4 mg
Fluoride	1.5 mg	1.5 mg
Folic Acid	400 mcg	1000 mcg
Inositol	75 mg	100 mg
Iodine	150 mcg	250 mcg
Iron	18 mg	45 mg

Magnesium	350 mg	500-1000 mg with calcium 1:2
Manganese	2.5 mg	5-10 mg
Molybdenum	15 mcg	125-500 mcg
Niacin	18 mg	100 mg
Pantothenic Acid	4 mg	100 mg
Phosphorus	800 mg	800 mg
Potassium	100 mg	114-500 mg with calcium 1:4
Pyridoxine	2.2 mg	50 mg
Riboflavin	1.6 mg	50 mg
Selenium	70 mcg	200 mcg
Sodium	1100 mg	3300 mg
Sulphur	?	500 mg
Thiamine	1.4 mg	50 mg
Tin	?	500 mcg
Vanadium	?	500 mcg
Vitamin A (beta carotene)	15000 IU	10000-25000 IU (Note: Excess is toxic. Vegetable based is non-toxic.)
Vitamin B12	300 mcg	100-500 mcg—3000mcg is still safe.
Vitamin C	60 mg	1000-2500 mg—6000 mg for a short time is safe.
Vitamin D	400 IU	2000-6000 IU—10000 max
Vitamin E	15 IU	400-1200 IU
Vitamin K	70 mcg	140 mcg
Vitamin Q (CoQ10)	30 mg	60-200 mg
Zinc	15 mg	50 mg—over 150 mg is harmful.

Herbs (See Chapter 7)

Vitamins

Vitamins and minerals are necessary for growth, function, and general health. We theoretically get most of these substances through the foods that we eat.

There are fourteen vitamins. Vitamins A, D, E, and K are fat-soluble and can be stored in the body. The other ten are water-soluble and have to be replenished.

Here are some facts about vitamins that you may not know:

- **Multivitamins** can help reduce the risk of cataracts, especially those containing vitamins C and E.
- **Vitamin A** can help improve eyesight, but it is fat-soluble and overdoses can cause problems. It is helpful for eye protection, healing of wounds, and immune stimulation. It can also prevent dry skin and aging.
- **B-vitamins** are all water-soluble and need to be replaced daily. Deficiencies can cause all kinds of disorders. B-vitamins are essential for the health of the brain, the eyes, the gastrointestinal tract, the hair, the liver, the nails, the nerves, the mouth, and muscle tone. They support methylation which prevents a rise in homocysteine levels in the body. Excess homocysteine is a toxic byproduct of the metabolism of methionine, which triples the risk of heart attack and causes other maladies such as Alzheimer's disease, dementia, depression, erectile dysfunction, kidney disease, osteoporosis, peripheral vascular disease, and retinopathy. B-complex deficiency in the body will show by cravings. People satisfy these cravings by turning to cake, candy, cookies, gum, ice cream, or other sugary desserts.
- **Vitamin B1** (thiamine) helps slow aging. It also aids circulation, digestion, and the production of hydrochloric acid in the body. It boosts energy and metabolizes carbohydrates.
- **Vitamin B2** (riboflavin) helps energy, growth, hair, mouth sores, skin, stress, and the metabolism of carbohydrates, fats, and proteins.
- **Vitamin B3** (niacinamide) helps the nervous system, production of sex and adrenal hormones, moods, circulation, the memory, the nerves, the skin, stress, and production of hydrochloric acid in the stomach.
- **Vitamin B5** (pantothenic acid) is an antioxidant that helps allergies, energy, nerve disorders, adrenal hormones, reduce stress, inhibit hair color loss, and prevent arthritis and high cholesterol.
- **Vitamin B6** (pyridoxine) helps allergies, arthritis, asthma, cancer immunity, cramps, hair loss, insomnia, numbness and tingling in the hands or feet, and the formation of homocysteine that attacks the heart muscle. It is also a mild diuretic.

- **Vitamin B9** is helpful for anemia, graying hair, and body repair.
- **Vitamin B12** (cyanocobalamin) helps absorption of food, anemia, balance, coordination, digestion, depression, energy, metabolism, moods, and nerves. Strict vegetarians require supplementation of B12 because they generally do not get enough protein. A deficiency in B12 may cause symptoms similar to those of multiple sclerosis.
- **Vitamin B15** is helpful for cell life, fatigue, and the liver. It can also control the craving of liquor.
- **Vitamin B17** (laetrile) contains natural cyanide, which is a poison being studied in the treatment of killing cancer cells.
- **Para-aminobenzoic acid** (PABA) is a basic folic acid and one of the B-vitamins found in B-complex. It has antioxidant properties that help protect the skin against skin cancer, sunburn, and ultraviolet rays. Some people can be allergic to this and care should be used.
- **Vitamin C** is water-soluble and necessary for many body processes including strengthening the immune system and warding off disease. Vitamin C is added to skin care products because of its collagen-stimulating properties. The antioxidant property of vitamin C is the reason it is helpful in the prevention and treatment of diseases, particularly colds and the flu. Cancer patients who are receiving radiation should not take vitamin C. If you are taking vitamin C, notify your doctor, as some test results can be altered.
- **Vitamin D** is fat-soluble. The body stores it; it is helpful for building bones, aids nerves, sleep, skin, and teeth. It is best used as a preventive. It benefits those persons undergoing chemotherapy, fighting colds and infections, and is essential to the formation of collagen. Before having any medical tests, be sure your doctor knows if you are taking vitamin D, as test results may be misleading. Vitamin D helps lower the risk of some types of cancer, heart disease, hypertension, multiple sclerosis, osteoporosis, and tooth loss. As many as one and a half million Americans have fractures of the hip, spine, or wrist that are osteoporosis-related. Your body produces vitamin D naturally when in contact with sunlight. Several hours of sunlight can produce up to 10,000 IU. Vitamin D is not actually a vitamin, but a hormone that works directly on the DNA of the cells and is necessary for the small intestine to absorb calcium. Low vitamin D levels have a strong influence on cell differentiation and proliferation and have been noted in persons with

osteoporosis. High ratios of aging symptoms, circulatory problems, insulin dependent diabetes, lipids, multiple sclerosis, obesity, and rheumatoid arthritis are noted in areas where vitamin D availability is low. Something to note about the possible importance of vitamin D is that, due to sun exposure, the occurrence of multiple sclerosis is almost non-existent in countries located near the equator. Ask your medical professional for a calcidiol measurement test. A minimum level below thirty-seven is an indication of vitamin D deficiency.

- **Vitamin E** is a fat-soluble antioxidant and when taken with selenium becomes even more effective. It can be helpful for blood flow, cholesterol, the eyes, fatigue, headache, the heart, menopause, muscle cramps, potency, and muscle cramps. Vitamin E also helps prevent rheumatoid arthritis (recommended maximum dose is 1200 mg), but don't take mega-doses without consulting a doctor; it could raise your blood pressure and interact with prescription drugs.
- **Vitamin F** is found in unsaturated fatty acids, essential for good health, helpful for the heart, nerves, reproductive system, and the skin.
- **Vitamin H** is water-soluble, essential for metabolism, helpful for growth, hair loss, mental health, muscles, and the skin.
- **Vitamin K** is produced in the bodies of healthy people and is necessary for blood clotting, normal function of the liver, the conversion of glucose to glycogen for body fuel, and to help peptic ulcers. Natural forms of vitamin K are nontoxic and safe, but synthetic forms can cause problems.
- **Vitamin P** is water-soluble, aids the cells, is helpful for asthma, bruising, gums, and resistance to disease. It works synergistically with vitamin C.
- **Vitamin Q** (CoQ10) is found in every cell in the body and functions as an antioxidant; however, the body makes less and less as you age. It is a vital nutrient used to produce energy and necessary for heart function. It is crucial in treating any degenerative neurological disease, especially Parkinson's.
- **Vitamin U** is used in treating ulcers, but very little is known about it.

Minerals

Calcium, chloride, chromium, copper, fluoride, iodine, iron, magnesium, molybdenum, potassium, selenium, and zinc are all important, each in their own way, as they contribute to growth and health.

Additional Supplement Information

- **Antioxidants** help the immune system fight free radicals and protect against aging and many illnesses.
- **Amino acids** are the building blocks of proteins and are necessary to break down fats for energy use. There are twenty-two known amino acids. Eight are called essential and cannot be produced by the human body. They must be either supplemented or obtained from foods. The eight essentials are isoleucine, leucine, lysine, methionine, phenylalanine, threonine, tryptophan, and valine.
- **Biotin** is produced in the body and promotes strong bone marrow and nails, healthy hair, and nerve cell growth. Deficiency of this is rare.
- **Calcium** is an essential component for bone density and heart functions. Calcium citrate supplements may be a natural way to restore bowel regularity.
- **Choline** is needed for gall bladder, brain, and liver function, lecithin formation, memory, and nerve impulses. It helps metabolize fat and cholesterol.
- **Chlorophyll** is a supplement that will help with dioxin, a potent carcinogen like PCB, and waste removal from the body. This is a big help to many body functions.
- **Cytochrome C** is an amino acid compound and is an energy stimulant that increases muscle performance.
- **Docosahexaenoic acid** (DHA) is a fatty acid. Low levels of this can cause aggression, Alzheimer's disease, depression, multiple sclerosis, and schizophrenia. About 60 percent of the brain is made up of fatty material and 25 percent of that fatty material is DHA. Humans cannot produce DHA, therefore it must be supplemented. DHA is found in breast milk, and breast fed babies tend to have a higher IQs than formula fed babies. Low levels of DHA in children are a major contributor to Attention Deficit Disorder (ADD) and Attention Deficit Hyperactivity Disorder (ADHD). DHA helps supply the brain with serotonin which regulates moods. Low levels of DHA may cause symptoms in multiple sclerosis patients such as: loss of coordination, muscular weakness, and speech and visual disturbances. These symptoms may be improved with Omega-3 fatty acids and DHA, which can be purchased from health food stores.

- **Evening primrose oil** is a supplement that helps supply the body with good fatty acids and is very important to hair, nerves, and skin.
- **Flaxseed** is a whole food with fiber and Omega-3 fatty acids. It is helpful for the prostate and prevention of breast cancer. It can also help promote healthy bowel functions and decrease the risk of diverticulosis that causes abdominal pain and cramping.
- **Folic acid** (folate) is needed for the brain, cell development, energy, and the formation of red blood cells. It is also important during pregnancy, as it can help eliminate birth defects of the spinal cord and brain. It can help lower the risk of homocysteine related diseases; 400 mcg is recommended daily with up to 5000 mcg for those with very high level of homocysteine.
- **Ginseng** is an energy stimulant and helps with the assimilation of vitamins and minerals. It is most effective taken on an empty stomach.
- **Glutathione** treatment, which is administered by IV, is an antioxidant that can ease depression, improve speech, mobility problems, and tremors, particularly in Parkinson's disease patients.
- **Homocysteine** is an amino acid. When their levels are too high, they are an indicator of deficiencies of critical vitamins. A high homocysteine level can lead to Alzheimer's disease. It is a good idea to increase consumption of fresh fruit and fresh vegetables to raise levels of B6 and folic acid in the body. A homocysteine level over ten is dangerous. If concerned, have your doctor check your level.
- **Inosine** is a nutrient to help combat fatigue. It increases the oxygen-carrying capacity of the blood, getting more oxygen to the muscles.
- **Inosital** is necessary to combat depression, vital for hair growth, prevents the hardening of arteries, and reduces high cholesterol.
- **Melatonin** is the hormone that induces sleep and used as a supplement is safe. Care must be used as too much may cause a reverse of the effective use. The pineal gland produces melatonin; as we age, it becomes calcified and its production decreases.
- **Nutraceuticals** are found in food or dietary supplements. They help the physiologic processes in the body.
- **Octacosanol** boosts energy and stamina; helps reduce heart stress, and can help in the rebuilding of the myelin sheath.
- **Omega-3, -6, and -9** are fatty acids that help reduce the pain and discomfort of arthritis and aid circulation; if needed, they can be added with supplements.

Omega-3, -6, and -9 help the body in the absorption of vitamins, along with helping ward off dandruff, dryness, eczema, hair loss, and psoriasis.

- **Phytochemicals** are produced by plants and give protection from a variety of diseases.
- **Phytonutrients** are found in plants. Beta-sitosterol, campesterol, and stigmasterol belong to this group. They are sterols or phytosterols and are similar to cholesterol, only they have fewer side effects. They are difficult to absorb. They increase the body's immune functions and help lower cholesterol levels. Sterol supplements help increase the production of disease-fighting T-cells and have similar effects to the drug cortisone without the side effects.
- **Propolis** is an energizer and a rich source of minerals, B-vitamins, and natural antibiotics. It can also stimulate the thymus gland and help the immune system, thereby increasing energy.

Fighting Aging

Protect your mitochondria, which are the energy-producing units in every cell of your body. Adenosine triphosphate (ATP) is a molecule in your mitochondria that glucose helps generate for protection from free radicals. Increasing your antioxidants will help protect the mitochondria. Alpha lipoic acid (50 mg/day) is an excellent antioxidant and is both water-soluble and fat-soluble. Vitamin E, CoQ10, and L-carnitine are also beneficial, as they will help curtail the aging process and promote younger looking skin.

Enzymes

Enzymes play an important role in our bodily functions. Enzymes are necessary to decrease inflammation, help remove waste products, improve circulation, reduce circulating immune complexes, speed tissue repair, stimulate immunity, and transport nutrients. Digestive enzyme supplements are taken to help digest food for assimilation. There are three main categories of enzymes for digestion:

- **Amylase** breaks down carbohydrates
- **Lipase** breaks down fats and oils
- **Protease** digests protein

Heat, long-term storage, pasteurization, pressure canning, and synthetic pesticides destroy the enzymes in raw foods. Age, prescription drug treatment, and stress deplete the ability of the body to produce enzymes. Illness interferes with production of digestive enzymes. Low body temperature (hypothyroidism) can be caused by an under-active thyroid and will cause poor digestion. Enzyme supplementation can help. Amylase, bromelain, catalase, cellulase, chymotrypsin, lactase, lipase, pancreatin, papain, pepsin, rennin, and trypsin are supplements that can be purchased at health food stores. Enzymes come in different combinations specifically targeting certain digestive problems.

Enzyme treatments are based on each individual; the theory of one size fits all is not true. Tests must be done on each individual to find out what is happening in his or her body. These include full range amino acid tests, hair analysis/mineral tests, histamine level tests, red cell analysis, and tests to see if you have enough calcium, magnesium, and potassium in your body.

CHAPTER 6
EXERCISE AND WATER

This chapter outlines different kinds of exercise as well as providing alternative ways to stimulate muscles. It also contains information on the importance of water. The material in this chapter was derived from articles, books, web sites, magazines, newsletters, and personal experience.

Exercise

As a rule, people who exercise are healthier than those who do not, yet only a small percentage of the population makes the effort. Many people think that their active lives give them enough of a workout, but unless one's work is physically demanding, it is safe to say that the activities of daily living will not keep a person strong and healthy. If you have ever been confined to bed for a few days, you know how stiff your muscles become. Muscles that are not regularly used tend to be sluggish when you do need them.

Exercise is very important for those of us with MS. Problems with coordination prevent performing some of the activities needed to keep the muscles toned. It is a good idea to check with your health care provider before you begin any exercise program.

No matter what exercises you choose, make a commitment, have fun, and fight boredom by adding variety. A good suggestion is to exercise three to five times a week for twenty to thirty minutes and never immediately after eating. Stretching and warming up prior to exercise is essential. It is also important to stretch and cool down after exercise to relax muscles. Know your limits and push yourself safely without going too far.

Exercising your heart and lungs along with other muscles is also important. You need to boost your metabolism. You can increase your metabolic rate by decreasing the amount of fat on your body and replacing it with muscle. Weight training is beneficial and should be started with small weights. It is a good idea to take a day off between weight-training sessions to give your body a chance to build new muscle.

People who exercise have a 30 percent lower mortality rate. Exercise increases fitness by about 25 percent after three to six months. It raises HDL cholesterol, lowers triglycerides and blood pressure, and improves insulin sensitivity.

Monitoring your heartbeat while exercising is important. Raising your heartbeat too high depletes oxygen from the brain. To see if your heartbeat falls within normal limits, use this formula. Subtract your age from 220 and multiply that number by 0.70 to find the low end of your heartbeat range. Multiply by 0.85 to find the high end. These numbers are the range for your age. It is best to check your pulse at your wrist or wear a monitor, as checking at the side of the neck is not as accurate. Normal range for a forty year old is 180 at the high end and 125 at the low end. The high end for a sixty year old is 160 with the low end at 111. The drop in numbers on the high end is one per year as age increases, and about 0.7 per year on the low end.

One of the symptoms of MS that develops over the years is muscle weakness. It is very important, especially for PWMS, to maintain a regular exercise routine. Some of the factors that cause muscle weakness are: misalignment of skeleton and deficiencies of vitamins, minerals, hormones, and enzymes.

Types of Exercise

There are essentially four types of exercise: aerobic, anaerobic, isometric, and isotonic.

- **Aerobic exercise** involves medium intensity for a long duration. It will increase your stamina and endurance. Examples are aerobics and long distance running.
- **Anaerobic exercise** involves high intensity for short bursts. This type of exercise is required for training athletes and uses up oxygen stored in the body. An example is running sprints.
- **Isometric exercise** is low intensity with more emphasis on toning. There is very little movement, but by putting a minor tension on muscles, it helps prevent atrophy. An example of this is trying very moderately to lift a chair you are sitting in. Other examples are pilates and mild yoga.
- **Isotonic exercise** is strenuously using muscles. This is the type used to build muscle mass and strength. An example is weightlifting.

Alternative Types of Muscle Stimulation

There are many ways to stimulate one's muscles: Swedish massage, reflexology, therapeutic massage, stretching, Tai Chi, trigger point, stress relief, deep tissue massage, acupressure, energy clearing, rolfing, and yoga. Here is more information on several of these activities:

- **Massage** helps loosen tight muscles and relax the entire body. It can help those who are not particularly active. It improves blood circulation, hastens the elimination of toxins in the joints, helps with the flow of energy, and circulates lymph (a coagulable fluid containing mainly lymphocytes and fats) with muscle movement. Stretching and relaxing is combined with relieving muscle pain or tightness by the elongation and relaxation of muscles. Normally, after a massage, you must drink lots of water to flush out the toxins in the body that are stirred up. Toxin build-up can result in poor health.
- **Therapeutic massage** is helpful for inactive people. They use this quite often in hospitals on bed-bound patients to help their muscles stay toned so the patient can still move around once they have left the hospital. This also helps particular forms of degenerative diseases such as arthritis and multiple sclerosis. A monthly massage is beneficial and rewarding.
- **Rolfing** is a very deep massage that has to be done in a series. In rolfing, someone can spend an hour just massaging your feet. For me, this experience was amazing and enlightening. Pictures prior to the first treatment and after the last (ten treatments total) had me standing up straighter; as compared to a picture on the wall, I was about two inches taller.
- **Tai Chi** is a Chinese exercise that improves balance and body awareness through slow, graceful, and precise movements while meditating. It has been effective in reducing chronic arthritis pain. This technique increases circulation and stimulates the repair of damaged joints and muscles. It is good exercise for older people because of its gentle approach.
- **Yoga** is an Eastern form of exercise and body relaxation used to relieve stress, increase endurance, tone muscles, and help the elasticity of the spine. It works by exercising all muscle groups with an emphasis on breathing. This can be done while sitting or lying on a floor mat. Yoga is beneficial both to your body and mind.

Water

Water is the most essential health-giving tool. Give yourself the gift of the best health you can achieve: drink lots of water. Water is nature's diuretic and cleanses your body. Chronic, unintentional dehydration is the root cause of many diseases. Increasing the amount you drink can help many health conditions. You should drink about two quarts of water daily unless you have kidney problems. If you drink water only when you are thirsty, then you are already in a dehydrated state. When you are dehydrated, your body produces histamines that prevent water loss through the lungs.

Your kidneys cannot function properly without water; if they don't have enough, their extra load is transferred to the liver. The liver's primary function is to metabolize fat into energy and dispose of waste.

Water retention—possibly caused by excess salt—may cause the feet, hands, and legs to swell. Drinking more water will force the excess sodium out through the kidneys. Muscles need water for proper tone, and water can help relieve constipation. Water is the key to fat metabolism: your body is physically unable to break down fat without it. Lack of water is a major cause of daytime fatigue. As you get older, your sense of thirst diminishes; hence you might not drink enough water, which can contribute to the development of diseases such as arthritis.

Approximately 70 percent of a person's body is water, and bones are almost 20 percent water. Blood is 55 percent plasma, and plasma itself is 90 percent water. The protective coating of the stomach is 98 percent water. Synovial fluid, the lubricating material of the joints, is mostly water. Drinking water restores the mucous membranes in the stomach that protect the walls of the stomach from hydrochloric acid. Hypertension's primary cause is a lack of water.

Water constitutes a major portion of protoplasm, which is a basic and necessary substance of plant and animal tissue.

Sewage and other poisons are found in water, and purification is required to make consumption safe. Many filtration systems are marketed and filtered water can be purchased. Tap water is generally not very healthy. Health professionals recommend drinking bottled or filtered water. Water filtered through a reverse osmosis membrane is best, as it removes most of the impurities. The quality of water you drink is important. It should be cool but not iced.

CHAPTER 7
SUPPLEMENTS

In this chapter, specific supplemental informational data was taken from one or more of the following sources: *The How to Herb Book* by Velma J. Keith and Monteen Gordon, *Nature's Choices* by Julie Aikens, *Herbal Products for Your Health* from Nature's Sunshine®, and *Shaping Up with Vitamins* by Earl Mindell R.Ph., PhD. For additional research, I recommend contacting health food stores or food supplement companies. As always, the Internet and bookstores are invaluable research tools.

Supplement Facts

If you are not taking supplements, you should be. Prepared and processed foods alone do not meet nutritional needs. It is not easy to find competent guidance about supplements. Most doctors have minimal training in nutrition, so asking your doctor about supplements might not be sufficient. Finding a path that you are comfortable with is a major job, but if you are willing to make the journey, it will be worth it. There will be signs along the way telling you if you are getting healthier.

In the rest of this chapter, you will find suggestions on possible sources for help in making your own educated choices. Make rational, economic, and beneficial choices. Start the journey: read, ask questions, and shop. Supplements do not show benefits immediately and usually have to be taken for approximately one to three months before results are noticed. If taken without any other drugs, no serious side effects are likely to result. Be open to going outside the box but do not just jump into something. Get a second opinion; ask those who have tried what you are considering.

Orthomolecular nutrition treats disease by either increasing or decreasing the intake of natural substances. The Internet has a lot of information, but everything you read is not necessarily true, so be wise and selective in your choices.

In the next pages, you will find some selections of informative material. There is a lot of information out there. Only a few supplements have been thoroughly and scientifically researched and tested. I have written about them from the assumption that they do what folk medicine says they will. You must make up your own mind about the effectiveness of any supplement listed here.

The following is not intended to provide medical advice, diagnose, prescribe, or replace the advice of a medical practitioner.

A Brief Glossary of Supplements and Possible Uses

Acidophilus helps replenish friendly bacteria in the intestinal system that caffeine, drugs, and stress deplete. It helps prevent skin eruptions caused by unfriendly bacteria. If your stomach hurts after taking antibiotics, which can destroy the good bacteria, it is necessary to replace the friendly bacteria with acidophilus.

Aloe Vera can be found in juice form and is used to help constipation, irritable bowel syndrome, and as an immune system stimulant. In gel form it has excellent healing qualities that can help give relief from abrasions, acne, bruises, burns, colic, colitis, cuts, eczema, fever blisters, insect bites, pain, and sunburn. It helps promote hair growth and is often used as a poultice.

Alpha-Lipoic Acid is an antioxidant that may be helpful for people with MS. It has been tested on animals and has been shown effective in suppressing some MS-like symptoms such as coordination and energy.

Arginine is an essential amino acid that helps increase insulin secretion. Taken with water on an empty stomach, it can help the release of growth hormones and help block tumor formations. It also helps increase nitric acid in the body which is necessary for erectile function.

Biotin is a water-soluble vitamin (H) in the B complex family. It is necessary for bone marrow, hair, nails, and nerve-cell growth. Most adults do not need to supplement biotin because their bodies produce an adequate supply.

Butterbur contains muscle relaxants and inflammation inhibitors that could greatly help asthma, gastric ulcers, menstrual pain, and particularly migraine headaches.

Choline is one of the vitamins in the B complex family. It is necessary for the brain, gall bladder regulation, liver function, nerve transmission impulses, and lecithin formation. It is a cleansing agent that helps the kidneys emulsify cholesterol and eliminate fatty deposits.

Colostrum is a fluid babies receive when nursing. It is rich in antibodies, immune boosters, lactoferrin, and peptides. Bovine colostrums are identical to the human form, and high doses are well tolerated by the body. It is useful in treating illness, particularly in older people. Sold in health food stores and it comes in capsules, lozenges, and as a powder. Take a low dose for maintenance and up the dose—double or triple—for infections.

CoQ10 is an essential enzyme and antioxidant that is necessary for the production of energy in every cell in the body. Effective in helping to protect the cardiovascular system, a deficiency may contribute to degeneration of the brain. Most Parkinson's patients are found to have low levels of CoQ10.

Curcumin is a spice that comes from turmeric. It contains potent antioxidants and its anti-inflammatory nature inhibits spoilage. The spice that gives curry its yellow color, it is used in nearly every Indian dish. Curcumin has been shown to help improve blood flow and has been noted to warm the hands and the feet. It might be the secret to lower the risk of Alzheimer's disease and MS because in India, where dietary levels are high, the rates of these diseases are very low. For increased absorption, find a product combined with bromelain or piperine.

Cysteine is an amino acid found in most proteins. It helps the body with bladder functions, helps keep the skin soft, and helps slow the aging process and the formation of wrinkles. It makes up a significant portion of the hair shaft and contributes to hair luster and the prevention of hair loss.

Dehydroepiandrosterone is a hormone that helps increase well-being, memory, and nerve impulses, and decreases fatigue. It also helps erectile function. If you can't find it in a health food store, a prescription is needed. A compounding pharmacist can fill the order.

Dimethyl sulfoxide (DMSO) is used topically to help reduce inflammation from arthritis as well as for chronic pain. It could help people with Alzheimer's, erthematone, Raynauds, scleroderma, and systemic lupus. It does, however, have an odor. Another product that is a derivative of DMSO is MSM. MSM is safe, effective, and does not produce the "rotten egg" odor.

Flaxseed is a good source of Omega-3 and Omega-6, the good fatty acids. It can help lower cholesterol and triglyceride levels. It can help reduce the pain, inflammation, and swelling of arthritis. It is best kept in a dark bottle or away from sunlight.

Folic acid is necessary for the brain, energy, and the formation of red blood cells. It helps keep artery-damaging homocysteine levels in check. It is important during pregnancy. Folic acid levels are related to vascular health. Your body must have the enzyme methylenetetrahydrofolate to metabolize folic acid. Supplementation injections of B12 can have folic acid added for additional benefit.

Glucosamine helps rebuild damaged cartilage and chondroitin sulfate.

Glutamine is an amino acid that can help increase your growth hormones. It can help the pituitary gland and assist the treatment of chronic diseases that involve muscle degeneration.

Glutathione is a water-soluble peptide. It is one of the best detoxifiers and helps protect the body from free radicals (foreign substances).

Goathead is a common weed. The herbal extract has been used for centuries and has been shown to help increase testosterone levels in both men and women. It can help increase endurance, energy, and muscle strength. It can help low libido and sexual dysfunction. It is not recommended for men with prostate or liver problems.

Interleukin 2 is a T-cell protein. It helps stimulate the production of T-cells and immune interferon. It is an antiviral protein and may be helpful in cancer prevention. It is not available as yet in the United States.

Oregano is an aromatic herb that is used for seasoning food. It has antibacterial and antifungal properties. It may be helpful for treating yeast infections when used in the appropriate strength.

Ornithine is an amino acid that helps the immune system. It helps stimulate the release of growth hormones that help insulin work.

Papain is an enzyme found in papaya which helps in the early processes of immune cell formation.

Peppermint oil can be used to help relieve irritable bowel syndrome and is safe for children to take for an upset stomach.

Phenylalanine is a water-soluble essential amino acid that is a natural brain supplement. Phenylalanine (L-PA) is an effective analgesic that helps chronic pain. It has been effective in the treatment of depression. L-PA tablets taken one hour before meals for a period of up to six weeks should be helpful. Afterwards, cut the dosage to one tablet at a lesser strength for a short duration to see if benefits continue. If not, be sure to consult your medical provider.

Propolis helps enhance the immune system and stimulate the thymus gland. It is a source of minerals, B vitamins, and natural antibiotics.

Selenium helps retard aging and helps vitamin E in its important body processes.

Soy products are full of phytochemicals necessary for lowering cholesterol. They help protect women against a build up of too much estrogen and men against prostrate cancer.

Testosterone is a hormone necessary for both men and women (in smaller doses) that is crucial to help sex drive and performance.

Zinc is necessary to help rebuild and repair injured tissues. It helps promote the healing of wounds and infections, and is helpful to combat colds.

Individual Herbs

Alfalfa is a natural source of vitamins (especially A and K) and minerals. It contains eight of the essential amino acids and is for arthritis, anemia, bursitis, cramps, digestion, healing injuries, the pituitary gland, and rheumatism.

Barberry acts as a diarrhetic in the liver and helps dilate the blood vessels to lower blood pressure. It is used for anemia, blood purification, constipation, diarrhea, gallstones, heartburn, pyorrhea, and sore throat.

Barley Juice Powder is a natural source of vitamins, minerals, amino acids, and enzymes, and is a nutritive. It helps protect the body from free radical damage and radiation.

Bayberry helps tone female organs and can help relieve menstrual, sinus, and adenoid problems. It's used for acne, bleeding, bronchitis, chills, colds, dysentery, enemas, mucus, the sinus, sore throat, the thyroid, and varicose veins.

Bee Pollen contains all known vitamins, essential amino acids, and many minerals, enzymes, and coenzymes. It is a nutritive used to help increase energy, reduce allergic response to hay fever, and increase athletic performance. It is important to start with a small amount and build up to a particular dose. There is no need to take large amounts as it regulates and stimulates. It is used for allergies, anemia, asthma, bowel control, depression, the hair, the heart, memory, the prostate, psoriasis, vitality, and wounds.

Bilberry Fruit (concentrate) helps eye problems: failing vision, poor night vision, glaucoma, cataracts, and tired, irritated eyes.

Black Cohosh has an estrogenic effect. It helps regulate the female cycle, relieve symptoms of menopause, stimulate contractions during labor, ease afterbirth pains, and relax muscle cramps and spasms. It's anti-inflammatory and antispasmodic. It helps break up mucus in the lungs and head. Taking too much can cause a headache. It's used for arthritis, the bowel, childbirth pain, coughs, dropsy, headaches, hysteria, insect bites, muscles, nervous conditions, uterine problems, and to stabilize estrogen levels.

Black Walnut is high in iodine, which is necessary for thyroid health. It is a muscle and nerve supplement, anti-fungal, anti-parasitic, and helps to balance sugar levels. It is used for athlete's foot, boils, cold sores, eczema, fever blisters, fungus, hemorrhoids, intestinal worms, lupus, poison ivy, skin rash, tooth enamel, and ulcers.

Blessed Thistle helps strengthen the liver and digestive system, increase appetite, improve circulation to the brain, purify the blood, and balance the hormones. It is used for circulation, cramps, fever, headaches, the heart, the kidneys, memory, menstrual problems, the spleen, and teenage acne.

Blue Cohosh helps regulate menstrual flow, and can be used as an emergency poultice for allergic reactions to bee stings. It is used for bladder infections, bronchial mucus, childbirth labor, colic, cramps, insect bites, rheumatism, spinal meningitis, urinary problems, vaginitis, and whooping cough.

Buckthorn helps regulate bowel control and is not habit forming. It is used for constipation, fever, the gall bladder, gallstones, gout, hemorrhoids, warts, and helps expel worms and parasites. It should not be taken during pregnancy.

Burdock helps skin and liver problems. It helps stimulate the flow of bile and purify the blood. Good for advanced cases of arthritis, it helps break down the calcification and reduce the swelling of joints and knuckles. It is used for acne, allergies, arthritis, baldness, bladder infections, blood poisoning, boils, cancer, chicken pox, eczema, hair loss, lupus, pimples, psoriasis, rashes, and urinary problems.

Butcher's Broom helps remove plaque build up in the arteries. It helps prevent blood clots and strokes. It also helps clean and tone the veins. It is used to help the prevention of heart disease, hemorrhoids, heavy legs, post-operative thrombosis, and varicose veins.

Capsicum-Cayenne helps promote circulation. It also helps increase digestion and absorption. It has been known to stop the bleeding of internal and external wounds. It helps arteries, arthritis, asthma, bronchitis, chills, congestion, colds, the colon, digestion, energy, the eyes, fever, hangover, nosebleeds, palsy, senility, shock, the sinus, sore throat, varicose veins, and wounds. It helps improve the elasticity of veins and capillaries, high or low blood pressure, and clear congestion.

Cascara Sagrada is a strong natural laxative that is safe even for children to use. It helps stimulate the bile flow, sooth nerves, promote sleep, and detoxify the liver. It helps prevent peristalsis (involuntary contractions) in the colon and is used for constipation, croup, digestion, the gall bladder, gallstones, hemorrhoids, insomnia, the liver, and the expellation of parasites.

Catnip helps digestive ailments, colic, digestive cramps, and gas. It is a good remedy for children. It has a tranquilizing effect which helps to relieve anxiety, insomnia, menstrual cramps, and nervous disorders. It is used for acid stomach, acne, colds, diarrhea, fevers, headaches, morning sickness, and nerves.

Cat's Claw – Una De Gato has alkaloids that help improve the gastrointestinal and immune systems. It may be helpful in treating AIDS, arthritis, cancer, Chron's disease, diverticulitis, gastritis, and irritable bowel syndrome.

Chamomile helps relax nerves, calm the stomach, reduce inflammation, cure colds and fever, and ease drug withdrawal symptoms. It can be used for children. It is used for appetite, asthma, the bladder, circulation, colds, dandruff, digestion, eyewash, fever, headaches, hysteria, insomnia, leg cramps, menstrual flow, the nerves, quitting smoking, and worms.

Chaparral helps rebuild new tissue. It helps as a blood purifier, especially in cases of arthritis and cancer. It also helps to rid the system of drugs. It is used for acne, boils, bursitis, hair growth, and muscle cramps.

Charcoal is used for first aid. It helps cholesterol reduction, diarrhea, intestinal gas, and insect bites. It also helps to prevent ingested poisonous chemicals from being absorbed into the system. (Consult poison control before use.)

Chickweed helps dissolve plaque in the blood vessels and promote weight loss. It is mildly diuretic and contains saponins which help break down fats and suppress the appetite. It is used for allergies, blood poisoning, the bowels, fatty tumors, hay fever, psoriasis, and scurvy.

Chlorophyll contains life-giving nutrients. It helps blood sugar problems and the colon. It also helps lubricate the ileocecal valve and stop growth and development of harmful bacteria. It helps accelerate tissue cell activity and re-growth. It is a natural blood builder that helps regulate calcium levels. It helps stop the growth of toxic bacteria, inhibit metabolic action of carcinogens, regulate bile movements, and remove toxic metals. It is used for anemia, body odors, the bowels, the breath, energy, hepatitis, hypoglycemia, the liver, the nerves, the sinus, the teeth, and toxins.

Comfrey helps stimulate new cell production, which grow new flesh and bones. It helps as an infection fighter and blood cleanser. The tea can be used for a douche for yeast infections. It is used for acne, allergies, anemia, arthritis, athlete's foot, the bowels, bursitis, the colon, digestion, fractures, hay fever, mouthwash, sores, swelling, and wounds.

Cornsilk is a mucilaginous and diuretic herb. It is used for bed-wetting, bladder and high blood pressure, kidney inflammation, painful urination caused by prostate gland problems, and water retention.

CoQ10 is an important nutrient in helping to treat cardiovascular disease, diabetes, and gum disease. It helps strengthen the heart muscles and is very helpful for all heart conditions.

Damiana is an aphrodisiac and helps restore sexual drive in men and women. It is used as a blood purifier and diuretic. It is used for depression, energy, hormone balance, hot flashes, impotency, infertility, menopause, nervous anxiety, Parkinson's disease, the prostate and reproductive organs.

Dandelion is a blood purifier and diuretic. It is used for acne, age spots, anemia, arthritis, blood purification, bowel inflammation, cramps, diabetes, eczema, energy, gallstones, hepatitis, jaundice, leg cramps, rheumatism, water retention, and weak digestion. It is high in potassium and one of the best liver cleansers.

Dong Quai is both a male and female tonic. It is used for anemia, angina, arteriosclerosis, dehydration, dry skin, migraine headaches, the nerves, stomachaches, and toothaches. It helps build the blood, increase fertility, regulate menses, relieve symptoms of PMS and menopause, and strengthen internal organs and muscles.

Echinacea Purpurea helps stimulate the immune system. It is an excellent infection fighter and powerful natural antibiotic. It is used for antiseptic, bad breath, colds, ear infections, fevers, the glands, lymphatic system, mouth sores, sore gums, and strep throat.

Evening Primrose Oil helps control appetite and assists the body in the breakdown of cholesterol, dietary fats, stored body fat, and triglycerides.

Eyebright is used topically as an eyewash. It is used for allergies, cataracts, conjunctivitis, coughs, diabetes, glaucoma, hoarseness, inflamed eyes, inflamed eyelids, pinkeye, and vision improvement. It is also used internally for upper respiratory congestion.

Fennel aids digestion. It is mild and helps normalize appetite and increase urine flow. It is used for appetite, colic, convulsions, cramps, gas, gout, headache, mucus, the nerves, rheumatic pain, the sinus, stomach acid, urinary problems, and as a gargle.

Fenugreek helps expel mucus and phlegm from the bronchial tubes. It helps soothe a sore throat and expel toxic waste through the lymphatic system. It is used for allergies, anemia, bronchitis, coughs, digestion, emphysema, the lungs, migraine headaches, the nerves, sciatica, tumors, water retention, and wounds.

Feverfew helps ease pain and prevent some types of migraine headaches. It helps prevent blood clots and may relieve the inflammation of arthritis. If taken on a regular basis, it helps to ease the frequency and severity of common headaches.

Garlic is a natural antibiotic that helps kill bacteria, fungus, and viruses. It helps protect against infection, prevent heart disease by lowering blood pressure, and prevent hardening of the arteries. It helps build endurance and boost energy. It is helpful in killing and expelling parasites. It is used for arthritis, asthma, cancer, cholera, circulation, colds, colitis, coughs, fever, high blood pressure, influenza, insomnia, parasitic diarrhea, the prostate, spinal meningitis, toothache, tuberculosis, tumors, warts, whooping cough, and yeast infections. It is also excellent for use in enemas.

Ginger is a remedy helpful for digestive disturbances, intestinal gas, nausea, and vomiting. It is used for bronchitis, cholera, circulation, colds, colic, colitis, constipation, cough, cramps, diarrhea, digestion, energy, motion sickness, morning sickness, and sore throat.

Ginkgo Biloba is very helpful for asthma, blood circulation, and dementia. It can be helpful to enhance longevity and memory. It can help with senility and vascular disorders. Care should be used if also taking blood thinners.

Ginseng, Korean is a stimulant that helps the body adapt to stress. It helps improve brain processes, increase energy, and balance blood pressure and blood sugar. It is a hormonal herb that helps prostate problems and some menstrual disorders. All forms of ginseng can be taken for up to six weeks, but then should be stopped for two or three weeks before starting up again.

Ginseng, Siberian is a milder stimulant than Korean or Wild American Ginseng. It is better for long-term use. It is especially good for men as it helps alleviate and prevent impotency. It is used for acne, age spots, asthma, cancer, colds, digestion, endurance, energy, lung, pituitary gland, prostate, skin, the stomach, and urinary problems.

Ginseng, Wild American is a stimulant with actions similar to Korean Ginseng but milder and less stimulating.

Golden Seal is a natural antibiotic, infection fighter, and immune stimulant. It helps improve digestion and clean the liver. It is used to help fight cholera, staph, strep, and Escherichia coli bacteria, and to lower high blood sugar in diabetics. It is used for bladder infections, the bowel, Bright's disease, bronchitis, cankers, chicken pox, colds, coughs, diabetes, douches, earache, inflammation, kidney infections, measles, mouth sores, mucus membranes, nausea, the nerves, the pancreas, the prostate, psoriasis, skin cancer, sores, spinal nerves, tonsillitis, typhoid, ulcers, and wounds.

Gotu Kola helps enhance circulation to the brain. It helps problems such as memory loss, mental fatigue, inability to concentrate, and learning disability. It is used for aging, blood pressure, brain function, depression, energy, the heart, senility, stamina, and vitality.

Guggul Lipid helps protect the heart, prevent blood clots, and motivate weight loss, and has been known to lower cholesterol by over 20 percent without dietary changes.

Hawthorn Berries are used to help strengthen and improve the tone of the heart. They help promote oxygen intake and circulation of the heart. They help dilate blood vessels and normalize blood pressure. They are a cardiovascular tonic and astringent. They are used for the adrenals, angina, arteriosclerosis, blood pressure, edema, energy, the heart, infection, insomnia, the nerves, and stress.

Hops is a calmative. It is used for abscesses, boils, the bowels, the digestive pains of a nervous stomach, fever, the heart, insomnia, intestinal cramps, the nerves, rheumatism, sore throat, toothache, tumors, and ulcers. It can be used as a sedative. It helps reduce excessive sexual desire and the desire for alcohol.

Horsetail has antibiotic properties. It is high in silica (a mineral important to the health and formation of bone, hair, skin, and nails) and can be used as a healing poultice. It helps the body use calcium. It helps kill and expel eggs of parasites and dissolve tumors. It is used for Bell's Palsy, the bladder, diuretic, the ears, the eyes, the fingernails, the glands, the hair, the heart, the kidneys, kidney stones, the liver, the nose, nosebleeds, osteoporosis, parasites, the skin, the throat, and urinary disorders.

Ho Shou-Wu is for longevity and fertility. It is used for colds, diarrhea, hemorrhoids, impotency, longevity, menstrual problems, and tumors.

Hydrangea helps pass kidney and bladder stones. It helps prevent build up of calcium deposits in the body. It also helps relieve calcium stones, bone spurs, and calcifications. It acts as an anti-inflammatory, diuretic, and laxative, thereby aiding kidney infections and arthritis.

Juniper Berries are a strong diuretic. They are used for water retention, difficulty passing urine, and bladder and kidney problems. They help strengthen the brain, memory, and optic nerves. They help kidney inflammation. They are used for the adrenals, allergies, bed-wetting, the bladder, colic, cough, cramps, diabetes, digestion, dropsy, gout, hypoglycemia, itching, the kidneys, kidney stones, memory, mucus, the nerves, the optic nerves, pain, plaque, and urinary problems. They are also used as a gargle.

Kava Kava helps soothe the nerves and relax anxiety, tension, and insomnia. It is used for the bladder in fungal and urinary problems.

Kelp is high in iodine, which stimulates the thyroid gland. It helps prevent goiters, boost metabolism, treat radiation exposure, and clear toxicity of heavy metals. It is high in sodium, potassium, and trace minerals. It is nutritive and can be used in place of salt. It helps regulate body temperature and build cell membranes. It is used for acne, adrenal glands, arteries, bursitis, colitis, endocrine glands, energy, hair loss, infection, menopause, morning sickness, nails, the thyroid, and tumors.

Lecithin is a phospholipid. It helps control the flow of nutrients and waste into and out of the cells. It helps break down fat. It aids the body with absorption of nutrients and is helpful as a neurotransmitter and for memory. It helps lower LDL (bad) and improve HDL (good) cholesterol. This is very important for people with MS.

Licorice Root is a natural form of estrogen. It helps strengthen the adrenals to produce cortisol (an anti-inflammatory hormone) and adrenaline (another body hormone). It acts as natural cortisone: anti-inflammatory and hormonal. It helps caffeine cravings, diabetes, dry cough, endurance, energy, fatigue, hoarseness, intestinal inflammation, sore throat, stamina, and voice muscles. It helps relieve ulcers and hypoglycemia by helping stabilize blood sugar levels. It is used for Addison's disease, the circulatory system, ulcers, body vitality, and as a laxative.

Lobelia helps allergies, angina, asthma, bronchitis, bursitis, colds, colic, convulsions, coughs, croup, emphysema, headache, hepatitis, insomnia, intestinal cramps, laryngitis, decongest lymphatics, muscle spasms, the nerves, pain, and pneumonia. In large doses it induces vomiting. It is antispasmodic. It's used for teething and toothache.

Magnesium helps with angina, chest pain, circulation, energy, headaches, high blood pressure, and muscle cramps. It helps relax nerves and artery walls to improve blood flow. When given intravenously, it helps strengthen the heart and improve survival rate after a heart attack. It is one of our necessary minerals.

Marshmallow is a mucilaginous herb. It helps soothe and reduce irritations in the digestive system, intestinal tract, urinary passages, and lungs. It's used for dry cough, irritated bladder, and inflamed kidneys. It helps lubricate joints against irritations and dryness. It is a nutritive and demulcent. It helps attract toxins and carries them out through the bowel.

Milk Thistle helps blood circulation to the liver and helps prostate enlargement, hemorrhoids, pelvic congestion, and varicose veins.

Mullein helps strengthen the lungs in chronic degenerative respiratory diseases. It is used for allergies, asthma, bronchitis, chest colds, croup, earaches, glandular swellings, lung congestion, rashes, sinus, swollen joints, and tumors. It rehydrates the lungs. It is high in iron, magnesium, potassium, and sulfur.

Myrrh helps promote development of white corpuscles. It is a natural antibiotic that helps clean and heal the stomach and the colon. It is used for antiseptic purposes, bad breath, bedsores, coughs, emphysema, the gums, leg ulcers, mouth sores, the nerves, the sinus, toothache, and wounds.

Nopal helps strengthen the immune system. It contains phytochemicals that help inhibit cancer growth. It has anti-inflammatory and diuretic properties, and also helps improve the utilization of insulin for adult-onset diabetes.

Olive Leaf Extract helps promote good health. It is a natural antibiotic for help in treating aches, anxiety, colds, concentration, depression, energy, fatigue, fibromyalgia, flu, fungus, moods, pain, and stiffness.

Omega-3EFA, -6EFA, and -9EFA are found in fish oils. They help with arthritis, circulation, and liver function.

Papaya helps relieve gas and a sour stomach. It is used for allergies, baby's formula, digestion, diverticulitis, gas, hemorrhage, parasites, stomachaches, and worms.

Parsley helps stimulate digestion and menstruation, improve appetite, increase urinary output and kidney function, lower blood pressure, and dry up breast milk. It is used for the adrenal glands, bedwetting, the bladder, the breath, cancer, coughs, fever, the gall bladder, gallstones, gout, kidney stones, mucus, the optic nerves, the pituitary gland, the prostate, tumors, and wounds. It can be used a laxative.

Parthenium helps stimulate the immune system. It is used for urinary tract infections. It is sometimes used as an adulterant to echinacea.

Passion Flower acts as a nervine and sedative to help relieve insomnia. It helps reduce muscle spasms and convulsions, and regulate the heartbeat.

Pau D'Arco – Taheebo helps conditions of fungal growth, athlete's foot, and candida. It has antibiotic properties that help treat viruses. It's used for AIDS therapy, arthritis, asthma, baldness, blood purification, bronchitis, cancer, colds, the colon, dizziness, eczema, fever, flu, gastritis, herpes, hernias, indigestion, impotency, infection, the kidneys, the liver, malaria, Parkinson's disease, the prostate, respiratory problems, scabies, the skin, sores, the spleen, syphilis, tumors, ulcers, and wounds.

Peppermint is good for the stomach and colon. It helps clean and tone and promotes relaxation. It can be used in place of aspirin. It's used for bronchitis, chills, colds, colic, colitis, diarrhea, digestion, dysentery, fainting, fever, flu, the heart, nausea, the nerves, vomiting, and ulcers.

Plantain is used as a poultice for boils, bruises, burns, carbuncles, insect bites, itching, mastitis bruises, ringworm, running sores, snakebites, and tumors.

Poke Root is an antibiotic that helps to heal inflamed kidneys and reduce liver congestion. It's used for blood cleansing, breast tumors, cancer, colds, goiter infection, liniment, drying mucus, the sinus, the spleen, the thyroid, and weight loss.

Psyllium Hulls is a mucilaginous herb. It helps absorb water to bulk and lubricate the stool. It helps constipation, diarrhea, draw infection and poisons from the body, and reduce cholesterol and blood sugar levels. It is used for colitis, digestion, diverticulitis, urinary problems, and as a colon cleanser.

Psyllium seeds have the same properties as psyllium hulls, but with a milder action. They are helpful for bowel irritation.

Purslane is used for canker sores, cold sores, herpes infections, and viral disorders.

Red Clover is a blood and liver purifier. It is used for acne, arthritis, boils, bronchitis, cancer, coughs, psoriasis, rickets, skin problems, spasm, tumors, and whooping cough. It helps relax nerves and strengthen the immune system.

Redmond Clay is not an herb. It comes in green, red, and white forms, with red being the strongest. It helps relieve pain and reduce swelling. When used internally it helps detoxify the body, clean the intestinal tract, and expel worms. Much care should be taken with use, as there are side effects. It is used for boils, detoxification, eczema, the liver,   and tumors.

Red Raspberry helps stimulate, tone, and regulate the female organs. It can be used throughout pregnancy to help relieve morning sickness and enhance lactation. As a tea, it is mild and has a pleasant taste and can be used to help stomachaches and bowel problems in children. It is used as an antacid and for childbirth after-birth pains, colds, constipation, coughs, diarrhea, digestion, fevers, flu, gastritis, labor pains, mouth sores, nausea, sore throat, and vaginal discharge.

Rose Hips are a rich source of vitamin C and bioflavonoids which help strengthen the immune system and healing. They are helpful as an infection fighter, a nutritive, and a stress reliever. They are used for arteriosclerosis, arthritis, circulation, colds, fever, and the kidneys.

Rosemary helps boost the body's immunity against cancer by helping inhibit cox-2 enzyme. It also is used in shampoos to help prevent baldness. It is used for baldness, colds, coughs, headaches, high blood pressure, nervous conditions, nervous headaches, nightmares, sore throat, and weight loss.

Safflower helps relieve digestive problems. It helps strengthen the liver and gallbladder. It helps break fevers by inducing perspiration and is a mild laxative. It is used for acid stomach, arthritis, colds, digestion, fevers, gout, kidney stones, and skin disease.

Sage (garden type) is good to cook with to aid digestion. The tea is good as a hair rinse to restore color. It also helps headaches and baldness.

Sage (wild type) is an astringent and antiseptic. It helps promote tissue repair and fight infection-causing bacteria. It's used for bladder, bronchitis, circulation, colds, coughs, dandruff, digestion, dyspepsia, hair tonic, the heart, hoarseness, impotency, the kidneys, laryngitis, the liver, the lungs, the nerves, pneumonia, sore throat, night sweats, and yeast infections.

Sarsaparilla helps purify the blood by strengthening the liver and the kidneys. It helps relieve arthritis and skin problems. It helps strengthen the reproductive glands (helping men increase low sperm count and women to have hormonal balance). It is used for age spots, aging, blood purification, boils, catarrh, diuretic purposes, eyewash, gout, hair growth, heartburn, hormone balance, impotency, internal inflammation, psoriasis, rheumatism, and venereal disease.

Saw Palmetto helps tone the male reproductive system by helping relieve symptoms of benign prostatic hypertrophy (BPH). It helps to enhance male sex hormones and weight gain, and aids respiratory and digestive weakness. It is used for alcoholism, arthritis, asthma, bronchitis, colds, diabetes, flu, glandular tissue, mucus, the nerves, the reproductive organs, and sore throat.

Scullcap has a calming effect to help sleep, circulation, and digestion. It is used for alcoholism, circulation, convulsions, digestion, epilepsy, fits, gout, hangover, headache, hysteria, muscle twitch, nerves, neuritis, rheumatism, smoking, stress, and the thyroid.

Slippery Elm helps absorb toxins from the GI tract and calm the digestive system. It is a contact healer and mild laxative, and is useful for diarrhea, especially in children. It is helpful as a nutritive food for sick children and the elderly. It is a demulcent. It is used for the bowels, colitis, the colon, constipation, cramps, diaper rash, diarrhea, digestion, diverticulitis, fever, hemorrhoids, herpes, hiatal hernia, hoarseness, kidney ailments, the lungs, mucus, rashes, sexual problems, sores, sore throat, ulcers, urinary tract problems, and wounds.

Spirulina is a helpful source of minerals, easily digested proteins, and vitamins. It brings a full feeling to those trying to lose weight. It helps provide essential amino acids and is a nutritive. It helps clear conditions of toxicity and fatigue.

St. John's Wort helps relieve depression. It is antibacterial, antiseptic, and antiviral, and helps repair nerve damage from injuries. It has anti-retroviral action. It also causes sensitivity to light, so avoid excessive exposure to light when using this herb.

Thyme helps remove mucus from the head, lungs, and respiratory passages. It has a soothing, sedative action. It is used for anemia, bowel difficulties, bronchitis, colic, cramps, and fever. It helps fight infections, expel worms, relieve gout, headaches, heartburn, infections, and insomnia. It helps soothe the lungs, the nerves, body odors, the sinus, the stomach, tumors, and wounds. It helps break an alcoholic habit.

Turkey Rhubarb helps the digestive tract and digestion. It helps relax the colon. It is used for problems associated with the alimentary canal, appendicitis, appetite, the colon, digestion, hemorrhoids, the intestines, constipation, purgative functions, and the stomach.

Uva Ursi is a strong diuretic. It is used to help treat incontinence and bladder and kidney infections. It helps to disinfect the urinary tract. It acts as a disinfectant, diuretic, and astringent. It is used for bedwetting, the bladder, Bright's disease, digestion, dysentery, gonorrhea, hemorrhoids, the kidney, kidney stones, the liver, lumbago, mucus membranes, the pancreas, the prostate, the spleen, and urinary organs.

Valerian Root is a popular nerve tonic and sedative. It helps insomnia, nervous tension, and anxiety. It is a nervine and soporific that helps to regulate the heartbeat. It's used for alcoholism, arthritis, the bladder, blood pressure, bronchitis, colic, colds, contagious diseases, coughs, drug addiction, epilepsy, fevers, headaches, heart palpitations, hypochondria, hysteria, insomnia, the intestines, menstruation, muscle spasms, pain, restlessness, and shock.

White Oak Bark is an astringent. It is used for diarrhea, hemorrhoids, and varicose veins. It helps a sore throat and bleeding gums. It helps produce antiviral and antimicrobial activity. It is used for bladder infections, bleeding, douches, fevers, gallstones, goiter, hemorrhoids, kidney stones, the liver, the lungs, mouth sores, nausea, pinworms, sores, stomach problems, and loose teeth.

White Willow is an analgesic that converts to salicylic acid. Salicylic acid is mild to the stomach and performs like aspirin without the side effects. It is used for arthritis, asthma, chills, colds, earaches, fevers, flu, gout, headache, sore muscles, the nerves, and pain.

Wild Yam is an antispasmodic and anti-inflammatory. It helps diarrhea, intestinal cramps, pain, menstrual cramps, and rheumatism. It has been used for birth control but does not contain progesterone.

Wood Betony is helpful for the nerves, the head, and face pain. It is used for asthma, bladder conditions, colds, colic, delirium, epilepsy, fainting, gout, heartburn, the liver, the nerves, and pain.

Yarrow is an astringent. It is helpful as a wound healer with antiseptic action to help stop bleeding and reduce pain. It is used for arthritis, the bladder, colds, diarrhea, flu, lymphatic congestion, and varicose veins. It is a good blood cleanser.

Yellow Dock is a blood purifier. It helps strengthen the liver and increase the flow of bile. It is used for skin rashes and jaundice. It helps improve assimilation of iron in anemia and skin eruptive diseases. It is used for acne, anemia, boils, the bowels, bronchitis, cancer, chicken pox, cough, energy, fevers, hepatitis, the liver, the lungs, measles, parasites, the skin, sores, and scurvy.

Yucca is a blood purifier and is anti-inflammatory. It has been used for arthritis and infection of the bowel.

Herbal Combinations

There are also herbal combinations available made up of natural herbs that contain nothing synthetic. They are intended to help relieve specific symptoms caused by certain health problems.

5-W helps induce and ease labor when taken during the last five weeks of pregnancy.

AG-X helps ease digestive disturbances, belching, bloating, gas, and stomach indigestion.

ALJ helps to expel mucus. It helps respiratory problems, allergies, coughs, chronic sinus congestion, and pneumonia.

APS-II (with white willow bark) is a pain reliever and is anti-inflammatory. It is used in cases of arthritis, headaches, menstrual cramps, and nervous tension.

Artemisia Combination is used for intestinal parasites. It is used for dysentery, giardiasis, hookworms, and pinworms. It is not recommended for long-term use.

AS (with Gymnema) assists in weight loss by helping to curb excessive appetite and sugar craving. Note: when chewed, Gymnema makes sugar tasteless.

BLG-X helps ease digestive problems, bloating, gas, and indigestion. It helps strengthen the liver and cleanse the blood.

BON-C helps speed the healing of damaged tissues, broken bones, cuts, torn cartilage and ligaments.

BP-X helps cleanse the blood and strengthen the liver. It has laxative and diuretic effects. It is used for problems such as arthritis, constipation, fever, jaundice, and eruptive skin diseases.

BRN-AV is a respiratory remedy. It is used for asthma, bronchitis, and cough. It helps to dilate bronchial tubes, expel phlegm, fight infections, and reduce inflammation.

C-X is a female corrective. It helps relieve menopause symptoms, hormonal imbalance, hot flashes, insomnia, nervous irritability, and sexual disinterest.

CA Herbal helps the body utilize calcium. It is used for broken bones, cramps, injured tissues, and spasms. It helps fetal growth.

Capsicum and Garlic with Parsley helps increase immunity and lower high blood pressure. It also helps circulation. The parsley helps mask garlic odor.

CC-A is an antibiotic, antiseptic, anti-inflammatory, decongestant, and expectorant. It helps the common cold, chills, fevers, headaches, nausea, and sore muscles. It helps ease symptoms of respiratory congestion. It is designed to help care for and prevent winter colds and flu.

CLT-X is an anti-inflammatory formula. It helps intestinal inflammation, colitis, diverticulitis, and ulcerations.

Cranberry and Bucha Concentrate is used for urinary tract infections and water retention because it has a strong diuretic action.

E-Tea is a blood purifier. It is a noted, traditional anti-cancer formula.

Eight helps headaches, mild inflammation, nervous system disorders, nervous tension, pain, and stress. It helps to reduce the cravings of people trying to quit drinking alcohol or smoking and taking drugs or painkillers.

Elderberry Combo is a natural antibiotic. It helps prevent colds and flu by helping to strengthen the immune system.

Elecampane helps fight intestinal parasites. It is used for amoebic dysentery, giardiasis, hookworms, and pinworms. It is also used for respiratory and digestive problems.

Energ-V helps energy and fatigue.

Energ-V Pack is a pack that includes Adapta-Max (only found in this pack), Energ-V, B-complex, and Proactazyme. It helps improve energy and stress response.

Enviro-Detox helps support the eliminative systems (the liver, lungs, kidneys, skin and intestines). It can be used regularly to help remove toxins the body absorbs from food additives and household and job-related chemicals.

EW is designed to be made into a tea and used as an herbal eyewash to help soothe dry, irritated, or itching eyes. If used internally, it helps upper respiratory congestion.

Eyebright Plus is high in luten, a carotenoid found in the eye that is important to eye health. It helps prevent blindness, eye diseases, and macular degeneration.

Fasting Plus helps relieve hunger and fatigue. It helps stabilize blood sugar and enhances elimination of toxins while fasting.

Fat Grabbers contain herbs high in fiber that help absorb fat and reduce cholesterol. They may help dissolve fatty deposits.

FC with Dong Quai is a general female corrective to help PMS, menstrual irregularity, and menopause. It can be used for long periods of time.

FCS II is a general female corrective. It helps PMS, menstrual irregularity, and menopause. It is more medicinal than FC w/Dong Quai and its use is recommended for shorter periods of time.

Fenugreek and Thyme is a decongestant and expectorant. It is used to help relieve sinus and lung congestion. It is helpful for sinus headaches.

Fitness Plus contains stimulants and adaptogens. It is used to help improve athletic performance, digestion, and circulation. It helps neutralize waste acids that cause sore muscles. It helps tone the structural system.

Four is a decongestant and expectorant. It is used for asthma, dry cough, mucus, and sinus headaches that accompany hay fever and allergies. It helps to clear, open, and relax the lungs.

FV is used to help settle the stomach during flu or vomiting. It helps fight infections. It is also helpful for motion and morning sickness.

Garcinia-Chi is a pack containing Energ-V, Garcinia Combination, and SF. It is helpful with weight loss.

Garcinia Combination is an herbal weight loss product. It helps decrease hunger, balance the blood sugar, and increase energy. It helps use long-chain fatty acids while preventing them from forming.

GC-X is used to help lower blood pressure, strengthen the immune system, and improve circulation and elimination.

GG-C helps provide energy by helping rejuvenate overworked glands. It helps a broad range of mental and physical problems, including jet lag, inability to concentrate, and fatigue.

Ginkgo and Hawthorn Combination helps improve circulation to the heart and brain. It is especially helpful for the elderly.

Ginkgo/Gotu Kola helps improve memory and circulation to the brain. It may be helpful for Alzheimer's patients.

Guggul Advantage is a pack containing Black Currant Oil, Guggul Lipid, High Potency Garlic, Mega-Chel, and Omega-3 EPA. It helps increase circulation and prevent heart disease.

Herbal Pumpkin helps cleanse the lower bowel. It helps to remove worms and parasites from the body. It is high in zinc and is helpful for prostate problems.

Herbal H-p Fighter helps fight spiral bacteria and helicobacter pylori (which scientists say causes ulcers). It helps relieve and heal inflamed stomach tissues.

HIGS II is helpful for earaches, infected wounds, low-grade infections, lymphatic problems, respiratory problems, and swollen lymph nodes. It is safe for hypoglycemics.

HS II helps strengthen the heart and circulatory system. It helps balance blood pressure, lower cholesterol levels, and prevent and treat heart disease.

HSN-W contains herbs rich in silica for healthy hair, skin, and fingernails. It helps keep the bones strong and flexible and strengthen the nervous system.

HVP is a sedative and nervine for poor sleepers. It helps relax muscles and reduce anxiety and stress.

HY-A is used to help hypoglycemics. It helps correct blood sugar imbalances, improve digestion, and stabilize the adrenal glands.

I-X helps supply iron in an easily digested plant form. It is a good supplement to help those who are anemic, fatigued, pregnant, or just generally weak.

IGS II is a natural antibiotic. It is used for colds, flu, headache, and lymphatic and respiratory infections. If hypoglycemic, take HIGS II instead.

IN-X is a stronger remedy than IGS II and HIG II to help with swollen lymph nodes and infection. It helps support the elimination and immune systems. It helps ear infections, flu, kidney infection, prostate inflammation, and tonsillitis.

JNT-A is an anti-inflammatory and pain reliever. It is used for arthritis, inflammatory conditions, gout, and lupus.

JNT-AV has diuretic properties and is used for arthritis. It helps build, cleanse, and heal degenerated tissues. It helps relieve inflammation.

JNT-Ease is a pack containing Flax Seed Oil, Glucosamine, JNT-A, Proactazyme, and Sulfate. It helps relieve arthritis pain.

JP-X is a diuretic and has antiseptic properties. It helps urinary and glandular weakness. It is used for weak sexual function, scanty urination, and water retention.

K is a diuretic formula that helps relieve water retention. It is used to help bed-wetting, bladder and kidney inflammation, and scant urination.

KC-X contains herbs high in iodine, which helps boost energy, clear congestion and lymph nodes, and strengthen the thyroid gland.

Kudzu/St.John's Wort (concentrate) helps those trying to stop excessive alcohol consumption. It helps block the metabolism of alcohol in the liver and helps fight the depression that comes with withdrawal.

LB-X is a mild laxative. It helps cleanse and tone the colon, reduce intestinal cramping, and increase digestive fluids.

LBS-II I is a stimulant laxative. It helps soften the stool and relieves constipation. It helps clean and tone the colon. It helps reduce gas and bloating. It helps improve digestion and the growth of friendly bacteria.

LH is for chronic weakness of the lungs. It helps thin and expel mucus. It helps to relieve asthma, bronchitis, and respiratory congestion.

LIV-A helps build the blood, increase digestion, and strengthen the kidneys and liver. It is used for age spots, liver diseases, and a sluggish gall bladder.

LIV-J helps rebuild and cleanse a sluggish liver. It is used for age spots and alcoholism.

Lobelia/St.John's Wort is used to help people stop smoking. It helps relax nerves and reduce nicotine cravings. It has anti-depressant effects. It helps strengthen the immune system and damaged respiratory systems.

Marshmallow and Fenugreek helps clear mucus and phlegm. It helps soothe irritated respiratory passages. It is used for bronchitis, dry cough, hoarseness and throat tickle.

Marshmallow and Pepsin helps break down undigested proteins. It helps clear the large and small intestines and increase the absorption of nutrients.

Men's Formula (concentrate) is for men to help increase male glandular functions, reduce prostate enlargement, and relieve urinary disease. It is high in zinc, a mineral males need for proper sexual function.

Morinda Citrifolia and Officianalis helps strengthen the immune system by helping increase white blood cell count. It helps arthritis, burns, cancer, joints, lowered immune response, inflammatory diseases, repair pancreatic cells, and wounds. It helps promote cellular growth and repair, and has anti-bacterial activity. It helps type II diabetes and brings an overall feeling of well-being.

Natural Changes is a pack with calcium, chaste tree, CX, flaxseed oil, magnesium, vitamin D, and wild yam. It helps aging women balance hormones. It helps ease symptoms of menopause and osteoporosis. It helps prevent heart disease and relieve stress.

NBS-AV is used to help treat diabetes. It contains gymnema that helps block sugar absorption in the intestines.

NF-X is a general female corrective that helps balance female hormones, infertility, menopause, menstrual irregularity, PMS, and urinary infections. It can be used during pregnancy. It is similar to FCS-II but is more of a stimulant.

P-14 contains diuretic herbs and is used to help support the pancreas of the diabetic. It helps lower blood sugar levels and cleanses the body.

P-X helps reduce prostate enlargement and urinary problems in men. It is also used to help diabetes and kidney or bladder infections.

Papaya Mint Chewable Tablets contain digestive enzymes. They help break down proteins. They help expel parasites and prevent gas and heartburn. They help improve digestion and stimulate hydrochloric acid production.

Pau d' Arco Power Pack contains E-Tea, Pau D' Arco, and SC Formula. It is used to help treat cancer.

PBS helps diabetics lower blood sugar levels. It helps strengthen the pancreas and contains cedar berries that help the body produce insulin.

PLS II is used as an instant poultice to help promote healing by mixing the capsule contents with water or aloe juice. The paste can be used on swelling, bites, stings, burns, and minor injuries. It can be used internally to help soothe intestinal irritations.

PS II helps to relieve prostate enlargement and urinary problems in men.

RE-X helps the body relax without dulling the reflexes. It is used to help anxiety, insomnia, muscle spasms, nervous disorders, and stress.

SC Formula contains reishi mushrooms and shark cartilage. It helps to fight cancer, boost the immune system, and prevent tumors.

Senna Combination is an extremely strong laxative and should only be used occasionally to help relieve severe constipation.

SF contains diuretics and mild laxatives to help with weight loss. It helps suppress the appetite, improve digestion, build energy, and break down fat.

SKN-AV is an herbal product for skin problems. It is used to help acne, boils, eczema, infection, inflammation, psoriasis, and ulcers.

SN-X is an alternative to over-the-counter antihistamines. It helps detoxify the body, improve digestion, and dry excessive sinus drainage.

Special Formula #1 is a cleansing combination that acts as a blood purifier. It helps cleanse the bowel and stimulate digestive organs. It is a glandular tonic and helps strengthen the liver. It is used for cancer or toxemia.

Stress Pack (with Nutri-Calm) is a ten-day pack that contains Hops Concentrate, Nutri-Calm, STR-J, and SUMA Combination that are nervines and adaptogens. They work together to help treat stress and nervous disorders.

STR-J is a nervine formula used for addictions, anxiety, Chron's disease, hyperactivity, muscle tension, nervous indigestion, nervousness, and stress.

SUMA (combination) is a pack of adaptogenic herbs. It helps to balance the body systems, strengthen the body's ability to cope with stress, enhance circulation to the brain, stimulate the immune system, and increase stamina and endurance.

Super Algae is a high nutritional supplement that contains all the amino acids, as well as carbohydrates, carotenoids, and trace minerals. It helps to lower cholesterol and build the immune system.

THIM-J helps strengthen the thymus gland and regulate the immune system. The thymus converts lymphocytes into T-cells to help fight invaders in the body.

Three is a supplement of minerals and vitamins. It is used for anemia, glandular imbalance, and weak digestion. It is helpful for pets and pregnant women.

Trigger Immune is a supplement to help with crabby, grumpy, or negative moods.

TS II (with Hops) contains herbs rich in organic iodine that help build the thyroid. It helps nervous stress that is common with low thyroid function.

U helps relieve ulcers and internal bleeding. It is also used for boils, slow healing wounds, and sore gums.

UC3-J is for colon care. It helps relieve inflammation of the digestive tract. It helps Crohn's disease, colitis, hemorrhoids, hiatal hernia, inflamed intestines, irritable bowel syndrome, and ulcerations.

Una de Gato – Cat's Claw helps build the immune system. It helps hormonal imbalances and intestinal disease. It can help relieve degenerative diseases such as arthritis and cancer.

Wild Yam & Chaste Tree helps regulate and balance the hormonal cycles in women. It helps reduce cramping, menstrual irregularities, and PMS.

X-A with Yohimbe is a tonic for male and female glands. It helps to increase erectile function, promote sperm production, and stimulate sex drive. It can help frigidity and painful menstruation in women.

X-A is a tonic for both men and women that can help stimulate sex drive.

CHAPTER 8
PHOTOLUMINESCENCE

The chapter explains photoluminescence, a treatment that uses infra-red light to purify the blood. Most of the information on the history of photoluminescence was provided by the book *Into the Light* by William Campbell Douglass, M.D.

History

Light has been used for over a hundred years to stimulate different forms of healing. Photoluminescence was used in hospitals for many years, but with our present day medical programs and drugs, it is no longer accepted by mainstream medical practitioners. There are very few clinics in the United States that offer this treatment.

Photoluminescence is also referred to as ultraviolet therapy or phototherapy. Ultraviolet lights have an antibacterial effect and have been used for many years to disinfect and sterilize a variety of things including medical equipment. Photoluminescence treatment has tremendous potential for the treatment of anthrax, as it has been used as therapy for bio-warfare in the past. It rapidly relieves paralysis of the bowel and eases allergic asthma. Most side effects of photoluminescence are very minor, like flushing of the skin and irritation. Photoluminescence should not be used for atopic dermatitis (eczema), lead poisoning, and Staphylococcus aureus (a staph bacteria infection), nor should sulfa drugs be taken along with treatment.

Ultraviolet Blood Irradiation Therapy (UBIT) or Ultraviolet Blood Irradiation (UBI) is currently FDA approved as a treatment for cutaneous T-cell lymphoma (a type of cancer). Photophoresis, also known as extracorporeal photochemotherapy, is a process of white cell irradiation that is being studied for treatment of autoimmune insulin-dependent diabetes, graft versus host disease, HIV-associated disease, multiple sclerosis, rheumatoid arthritis, systemic sclerosis, and systemic lupus erythematosus. Electromagnetic fields combined with light help benefit the autonomic nervous system. Anyone interested in researching the scientific knowledge has volumes of data to observe from works that have been published over the last hundred years.

Benefits

Photoluminescence is used to kill infections—viral, fungal, bacterial, and toxic—in the blood. It helps increase red and white cell count and platelets, oxygen and protein content in blood, cell permeability, and vitamin D levels. It stimulates the body's own enzyme and immune systems to help cure diseases by killing infectious organisms and inhibiting bacteria growth. The blood's oxygen-combining capabilities and cortisone molecules are activated; toxins and viruses are inactivated. It helps to lower blood pressure and blood sugar levels, clear up bowel problems, and calm the nervous system and an overactive thyroid gland. This treatment can be beneficial to post-operative infections. Blood cells can be sensitized and antibodies can be made photoactive which may help autoimmune diseases. The chemical 8-Methoxypsoralen (8-MOD) in combination with UBI may help in the treatment of psoriasis. Studies are being done using this as treatment for multiple sclerosis. However, it should be noted that over-dosage could cause depression.

Photoluminescence has been used on patients with AIDS, allergies, arthritis, asthma, blood poisoning (septicemia), botulin, botulism, bronchitis, cancer, cerebral thrombosis, CMV, ear-nose-throat diseases, flu, gingivitis, heart disease, hepatitis, herpes, influenza, peritonitis, viral pneumonia, polio, rabies, sinusitis, staph, strep, tetanus, and tuberculosis.

Minor illnesses seem to respond well to occasional use of 10 ccs of blood being treated twice in one day. More serious illnesses may require treatments every five days over a few weeks using 1.5 ml of blood per pound of body weight. The treatment may be used daily with complete safety.

Treatment Procedure

Photoluminescence treatment involves the use of a sterile IV unit through which blood is removed from the vein and passed under ultraviolet light into a container. The process is then reversed and the blood is again passed under the light as it is returned to the body. The blood is never exposed to air during the process. However, the entire blood supply is activated and becomes an effective tool used to treat many viral and bacterial diseases. What does the treatment actually do? From my personal experience, I believe it improves the quality of the blood.

After having a Dark Field Blood Test, where they take a drop of blood and magnify it to evaluate the contents, they found 30 percent of my red blood cells were on their sides and inactive and there were very few white blood cells. I could see this for myself on the monitor. Seeing the results prompted me to try photoluminescence. After five treatments, I had another Dark Field Test. To my surprise, all red cells were free-floating and very active and there were many white blood cells. The technician was amazed. There was no physical mobility improvement.

Because this process kills bacteria, both good and bad, it is necessary to replenish the good stuff. This is usually done at the same time through another IV. This will most likely not be covered by insurance, and the cost of a treatment is approximately $300. Photoluminescence requires very few pieces of equipment and only a small amount of blood (200 ccs) needs to be exposed to ultraviolet light to energize the body's immune system. I have had a total of eleven treatments of photoluminescence; seven were performed years ago and four within the last few years.

Each clinic did the treatments differently. The first clinic put a butterfly needle in my left arm with a tube connected to a machine that pumped the blood out of the vein, through the ultraviolet light source of the machine, and into a sterile sealed glass container. Simultaneously, another butterfly needle and IV with vitamins and minerals (also called an Immune Boost) was being infused into the right arm. Once the container reached 200 ccs of treated blood, the pump was reversed and the blood passed once again through the ultraviolet light back into my arm. The procedure took approximately two hours.

The second set of treatments was performed by a slightly larger needle with two ports, one of which had a shut-off clamp. An IV bag of diluted hydrogen peroxide solution along with vitamins and minerals was connected to the port that could be shut off. After this IV had dripped down to approximately 10 percent, the tubing was placed in the ultraviolet light machine and a syringe at the far end was connected to the other port. The clamp was closed, and by withdrawing the plunger on the syringe, approximately 50 ccs of blood was slowly withdrawn through ultraviolet light. At that time, the plunger was depressed and the blood once again passed through the light. This procedure was repeated a few times (three minimum, five maximum). All the blood was re-inserted back into my arm. The tubing was disconnected and the clamp was re-opened to allow use of the remainder of the hydrogen peroxide IV solution. The entire process took approximately two hours.

CHAPTER 9
Bio-oxidative Therapies

This chapter explains the importance of oxygen, hydrogen peroxide, and ozone. Two books provided most of the information on hydrogen peroxide and ozone: *Hydrogen Peroxide Medical Miracle* by William Campbell Douglass and *Oxygen Healing Therapies* by Nathaniel Altman.

Oxygen

Oxygen is necessary for life and increases your chances of maintaining good health. The oxygen content in the air has been decreasing since the industrial revolution when it was at 32 percent. In the beginning of the twentieth century, it dropped to 24 percent; today, it is at about 21 percent. In larger cities and industrial areas, it can be as low as 10 percent. Life may not be able to exist if the percentage falls below 7 percent. The following treatments will add oxygen to a person's body.

Hydrogen Peroxide

History

Hydrogen peroxide is a molecule (H2O2) that is very sparse in nature. Traces are found in rain and snow, and yet it is found throughout a person's body. Estrogen, progesterone, and thyroxine production depend upon it. It helps to regulate body sugar, and is necessary for the immune system to work correctly. Hydrogen peroxide is generated by vitamin C that in turn protects, builds, and strengthens many body parts, including the heart. However, ingesting full-strength hydrogen peroxide or its vapor can be fatal. Hydrogen peroxide in a pure state is toxic; in a diluted form, it acts as a purifying agent.

Benefits

Hydrogen peroxide treatments have many benefits and only a few will be mentioned here. First, and probably most important, is the enhancement of one's own immune system. Hydrogen peroxide breaks down into water and oxygen once in the blood stream and stimulates the production of white blood cells. Bio-oxidative therapies stimulate the production of the white blood cells necessary to fight infection, increase oxygen delivery from the blood to the cells, and inhibit the growth of tumors. It stimulates the heart and thyroid and helps circulation. Treatments are very helpful in treating allergies, arteriosclerosis, asthma, bacteria, Bell's Palsy, botulism, bronchitis, cancer, candidiasis, chronic fatigue, chronic lung disease, chronic pain, Crohn's disease, Epstein-Barr, emphysema, flu, fungus, gangrene, herpes, infections, influenza, lupus, migraine headaches, multiple sclerosis, parasites, Raynaud's disease, rheumatoid arthritis, shingles, sinusitis, viruses, and yeast. It has destroyed cancerous tumors and been known to expel debris from the lungs. It also speeds the healing of wounds.

A series of treatments on a weekly basis may be needed for most serious diseases. One or two treatments will usually clear up a cold or flu. Treatments can be daily or spaced a day apart. Hydrogen peroxide (one treatment per week), along with chelation (two treatments per week), has helped angina pectoris, blocked arteries, and peripheral artery blockage in the legs. Ten weeks of treatment should be the minimum. There are some possible side effects and hydrogen peroxide will not help diseases such as carbon monoxide poisoning and chemical toxic shock.

Treatments

Treatments of hydrogen peroxide combined with other agents such as B complex, B12, CoQ10, copper, DMSO, EDTA, magnesium, minerals, photoluminescence, and vitamins (except vitamin C) target specific conditions. Hydrogen peroxide stimulates the production of T-helper cells that cause white cells to make interferon.

Oral hydrogen peroxide is also available. This is inexpensive, but there are many side effects and precautions must be considered. Dosages are not very predictable and reaction in the body varies greatly. Free radicals can be formed with stomach acids. A safe dosage is to not exceed ten drops of 3 percent food grade hydrogen peroxide. Some commercial brands contain a high content of lead, so the Regent grade should be used when taking   it orally.

Oral hydrogen peroxide is not the treatment of choice by most practitioners familiar with hydrogen peroxide therapy and is not as effective as IV treatments. A 3 percent hydrogen peroxide solution can be purchased in pharmacies and grocery stores for the disinfection of wounds and skin rashes and, when diluted, to cleanse food.

Potential side effects from hydrogen peroxide IV therapy are rare, as it is well tolerated by the body. The most common is vein inflammation (a red streak up the vein). There are two types of red streak: one is harmless and lasts twenty minutes; the other indicates vein inflammation, signaling that the needle position should be moved. Other side effects can include slight chest sensation or chills and is corrected by slowing down the infusion.

Another side effect is the Herxheimer Reaction, a short-term immune reaction due to the liberation of endotoxins or antigen substances, which is a good sign that the body is reacting satisfactorily to the expellation of toxins. The Herxheimer Reaction consists of migratory aches, chills, diarrhea, headaches, and nausea. This condition, if it occurs at all,   is temporary.

Another possible side effect is that hydrogen peroxide intensifies the anti-coagulant action of the drug Coumadin; therefore, the dosage of the drug might have to be reduced. If you are healthy and get a treatment, it is not harmful; you might just perk up.

Treatment Procedure

A typical infusion consists of the insertion of a butterfly IV needle into an arm vein, after pulse, temperature, and blood pressure have been taken. After securely taping the butterfly, it is connected to the tubing from the IV bag. The bag contains a much diluted hydrogen peroxide solution (0.0375 percent) mixed with saline or pure water. Vitamins and minerals can also be added to the solution. The recommended time for 250 cc is ninety minutes. A sterile cotton batten applied with pressure to the injection site of the butterfly needle usually prevents any after effects of localized swelling or inflammation of the vein. My latest series of treatments have been slightly different. The bags have been 200 ccs of pure water with 3 ccs of 3 percent hydrogen peroxide over seventy-five minutes with no pulse or temperature taken. I have had no problems.

Hyperbaric Oxygen Therapy

Hyperbaric oxygen is a treatment that involves flooding the body with massive amounts of oxygen in a pressurized environment. The patient sits in an enclosed chamber and oxygen is forced into the tank. This stops infections and encourages new tissue growth. This process is very common in treating "the bends" (a condition known to deep-water divers). People who have suffered a stroke will find it very beneficial. This therapy is also being used on some MS patients with noticeable benefits.

Ozone

Treatment Benefits

In a pure state, ozone is toxic. However, in a diluted form, it acts as a purifying agent. Ozone kills microbes, molds, and viruses; it has been used to help treat persons with candida albicans, cancer, chronic bacterial diarrhea, Crohn's disease, cytomegalovirus, E. coli, Epstein-Barr, herpes, hepatitis, HIV, inflammatory bowel disorders, pesticides, Salmonella, staph, strep, and ulcerative colitis. Ozone can inactivate and destroy toxins by oxidizing them. It should not be inhaled, and if it is, it can lead to emphysema, as lung tissue is sensitive. Bottling companies use ozone because it is a powerful disinfectant. Dentists may use diluted ozone to control bleeding, cleanse wounds, and promote healing. At the present time, there is no known way to encapsulate ozone for public sale.

Treatment Procedure

Another method of adding oxygen to the body is using an ozone generator, where oxygen is infused into the blood. This requires a special technique and needs very careful monitoring to prevent the possibility of a bubble forming and causing a blockage. There are also portable ozone generators that purify water by killing bacteria, parasites, viruses, and microorganisms that cause bad taste and odor in water. The ozone machine, when plugged into an AC outlet, emits ozone through a tube that leads to a container of water. Drinking this water may cause an energy boost.

If the body's process for oxygenation is weak, a toxic build up can cause dullness, fatigue, and sluggishness. Bio-oxidative therapies, like hydrogen peroxide and ozone, are non-patentable and relatively inexpensive, yet they have been effective in treating chronic and degenerative diseases.

Stabilized Oxygen Supplements

NASA developed the oxygen stabilizing process. Early oxygen supplements bonded oxygen atoms to chlorine salts. The latest process dissolves mono-atomic oxygen molecules in water. This new form of oxygen supplement is a liquid and is on the market. Information can be found by contacting the World Health Group.

CHAPTER 10
Chelation

This chapter explains the history, process, and benefits of chelation. The information in this chapter was derived from a few sources: *Forty Something Forever* by Arline and Harold Brecher, and the monthly newsletters *Second Opinion* by William Campbell Douglas, M.D. and *Health And Healing* by Julian Whitaker, M.D.

History

In 1893, a French-Swiss chemist, Alfred Werner, started research on what we now call "chelates" and won the Nobel Prize for his work. He wrote several books and over a hundred technical papers explaining how metals bind to organic molecules, forming the basis for chelation.

The first uses of chelating were commercial: electroplating and the removal of unwanted metals in the production of paint, rubber, petroleum, and other products and processes. Citric acid was first used for this. During the days of Hitler, the Nazi Party found a synthetic calcium-binding additive that would combine with metal impurities and keep stains from forming when mineral-hardened water reacted with dyes. In 1935, they developed ethylene diamine tetra-acetic acid (EDTA).

In the early 1950s, workers in a battery plant in Michigan were diagnosed with lead poisoning. The doctor treated them with EDTA, and not only did they get well, but they also noticed relief from chest pains, a symptom related to arteriosclerosis (hardening of the arteries). The treatment improved kidney function, arthritis, Parkinson's disease, and blood circulation. Chelation is now the treatment of choice for lead poisoning. EDTA was found to be less expensive and more effective than the citric acid that was previously used.

Chelation is a therapy that removes heavy metals (except mercury), calcium build up, and blockages in the blood system. The synthetic protein EDTA is a common ingredient found in many household items. It is especially common in water softeners.

Over five hundred thousand people have used chelation therapy in the last thirty years, but only 1 percent of the population in America has heard of it. About 80 percent of people using chelation were introduced to it by word of mouth. Only 1 percent of patients were informed by their doctors that the treatment was available.

Thousands claim to have been cured by chelation. The U.S. Government Office of Technology stated that chelation has been proven effective in lab tests. A FDA study of EDTA for arterial disease was started in 1985, but with the birth of open-heart surgery, the study was put on hold.

Benefits

Chelation therapy has a powerful disease reduction factor. EDTA chelation has an affinity for binding with heavy metals in the body and allowing them to be passed off in waste. These heavy metals cause serious damage to organs and the circulatory system. A zero level of aluminum, lead, and mercury is ideal.

How do we get these free radicals inside our bodies? There are many ways, such as: amalgam fillings, chemical additives, drinking impure water, consuming foods with unsaturated processed oils, radiation from television, inhaled toxic chemicals, smoking, and inhaling second-hand smoke.

As beneficial as chelation may be, chelation alone will not guarantee the prevention of a heart attack or stroke. Heart disease is the number one cause of death in America.

Warning signs of a heart attack are: chest discomfort, fainting, fullness, nausea, chest pain or pressure, and shortness of breath. Warning signs for symptoms that could lead to a stroke are: balance problems, confusion, loss of coordination, dizziness, face numbness or weakness, sudden headaches, and trouble seeing, speaking, or walking.

The list of benefits from chelation include:

- a downgrade in Alzheimer's disease symptoms
- a reduced need for diuretics
- better skin color
- emotional well being
- fewer wrinkles
- improved blood circulation
- some relief from impotence
- improved psychological thought
- improved senses of vision, hearing, and taste
- increased blood flow to the brain
- increased nail and hair growth
- lessened varicose vein pigmentation

- lightened age spots
- lower cholesterols in the liver
- lower blood pressure
- lower insulin requirements in diabetics
- lower blood cholesterol
- mental and memory improvements
- normalized weight
- reduced allergic symptoms
- some alleviation of Chronic Fatigue Syndrome
- some relief from leg cramps
- stronger nails

Chelation therapy can reduce the possibility of death by helping to clear heavy metals and toxins from the blood. High blood pressure causes a loss of calcium and a weakening of bone structure. Bypass surgery will not cure your disease. Records indicate that 5 percent to 10 percent of heart bypass surgery patients suffer a heart attack immediately following surgery, and 20 percent have neurological damage. Mental impairment, or the chance of it, can be caused by a lack of oxygen to the brain during surgery that might have been prevented if the surgeons had used hydrogen peroxide treatments prior to surgery.

People who have had bypass surgery should live longer, but research does not substantiate this. *Internal Medicine News* says symptom relief is short lived, and 30 percent to 50 percent of patients have a recurrence of symptoms within the first year. In comparison, there have been less than thirty EDTA related deaths verses eighteen thousand deaths as a consequence of bypass surgery, although more people have had bypass surgery. Heart bypass surgery is over-prescribed and a high-risk procedure.

There are other high-risk, invasive procedures used to treat artheriosclerosis. Balloon angioplasty involves the insertion of a balloon tipped catheter through the femoral artery to the site of blockage, where the balloon is inflated with fluid, stretching the passageway. Angiography, a pre-surgical x-ray technique, is used to detect blocked arteries. About three hundred thousand patients per year use this technique, which allows them to view the blockage. Atherectomy is a surgical procedure to open blocked arteries or veins by removing plaque with a catheter. Directional atherectomy uses a catheter with a cutter that shaves off the plaque and then removes it. Other treatments include transmyocardial revascularization (laser heart surgery), heart puncture, and artery stints. Heart bypass surgery is a six billion dollar a year industry, and heart surgery is a twenty-six billion dollar industry.

Bypass surgery bypasses a small segment of diseased vessel. EDTA helps clear the entire arterial system. Bypass is hazardous, expensive, and requires hospitalization. EDTA is relatively inexpensive, pain free, safe, effective, and convenient, but takes time and repeated treatments.

Hospitals can be a risky place to go. There have been cases of poor monitoring, improper blood transfusions, improper use of technological equipment, defective equipment, and anesthesia mishaps. Ten thousand deaths are reported each year from anesthesia administration. Out of thirty-five million Americans hospitalized each year, two million get sicker. Over one hundred thousand hospital-originated, infection-related deaths occur annually. In a report by the American Medical Association, sixty thousand to one hundred and forty thousand deaths a year are the result of prescription drugs.

Treatment Procedure

EDTA is a synthetic amino acid that is delivered intravenously. EDTA helps drastically to clear obstructed blood vessels. It provides symptom relief and minimizes the disease process. It combats hardening of the arteries that cause heart attack and strokes. EDTA has a particular affinity for toxic metals such as: aluminum, calcium, chromium, cobalt, copper, iron, lead, and zinc. When EDTA combines with such substances in the body, the metals lose their physiologic and toxic properties, and are excreted in body waste.

Blood platelet stickiness is the problem. Folic acid and vitamin B12 help your body detoxify excess homocysteine accumulation that causes thickening of the blood. Wine and moderate alcohol intake tends to thin the blood. Many new health practitioners have abandoned drug and surgery centered practices and made the switch to non-invasive remedies like chelation.

A small butterfly needle is inserted into an arm vein, and a bag with EDTA in a solution is infused into the blood. A full chelation takes three to four hours. A half chelation takes one to two hours.

The benefits of half chelation are nearly the same as full, and so I have chosen to receive only half chelation on a monthly basis as maintenance for protecting my heart and blood circulation. After having chest pains which led to hospitalization in 1995 and a subsequent balloon angioplasty, I did full chelation weekly for six months and then went to twice monthly before the present schedule of once a month. Since insurance does not normally cover chelation, it was also a matter of cost.

Calcium EDTA

Recently, there has been a new protocol for IV and oral EDTA chelation. It involves a direct push of Calcium EDTA of 50 mg per kilogram (not more than 3 gms) of body weight. This is given by an infusion, with no dilution, which lasts one to two minutes. These pushes can be administered two to three times a week depending on the patient's need for detoxification. This method of chelation has a much greater ability to penetrate deep into tissues to reach stored deposits of heavy metals and plaque. This treatment has been used in Europe for over thirty years with an 80 percent to 90 percent reduction rate noted in cancer and heart attack patients. One of the greatest benefits of Calcium EDTA is its ability to also detoxify mercury, as well as the other heavy metals.

This treatment can be given with other IV therapies as long as this is the final one. A side effect may be temporary weakness. Patients with known renal insufficiency should have a lower dose of the parenteral EDTA.

Other Treatments

Provocative urine and fecal minerals tests will indicate to a patient the increased burden of heavy metals in the body. These tests, along with hair analysis, are a good indicator of toxins and heavy metals.

There are many drugs such as antiarrhythmics, anticoagulants, antihyperlipidemics, beta-blockers, calcium-channel blockers, diuretics, nitrates, and vasodilators that are used to treat heart patients. Some of these drugs actually increase the risk of death.

Aspirin has probably been the most beneficial drug for people with angina. It can reduce the possibility of death after a heart attack by as much as 10 percent. If taken during a heart attack, the mortality rate is reduced by about 30 percent. On the down side, aspirin causes an increase in strokes and reduces blood platelet clotting. It can cause macular degeneration, block production of certain beneficial prostaglandins, and is linked to kidney and liver damage.

Beta-blockers inhibit the heart's ability to respond to epinephrine and adrenaline, which stimulate pulse and blood pressure. They are meant to lower blood pressure and ease pain. If a person stops taking them, it should be done gradually and under a doctor's care.

Another non-surgical therapy to consider for circulation improvement is Enhanced External Counterpulsation (EECP), which pumps blood from the legs to the heart, creating pathways around blockages, thereby improving angina.

Diet change, exercise, and supplementation are also necessary. Stopping smoking, reducing fat and sugar consumption, and increasing the intake of antioxidants will give your arteries a chance to recover and mend.

Other Chelating Agents

DMPS is specific mercury chelator and is relatively inexpensive. Recently, the DiSodium EDTA used in chelation was deemed able to adhere to some metals, but not mercury. Very recently Calcium DiSodium EDTA has been used with positive results for reducing mercury levels in the body. With DMPS, the infusion time is much quicker, and is not caustic to veins when infused in fifteen to thirty minutes. It also chelates both lead and mercury. These chelating agents, such as dimercaprol, EDTA, and penicillamine, bind strongly to heavy metals that are then usually excreted in the urine.

CHAPTER 11
Miscellaneous Alternative Treatments

This chapter describes a number of different treatments, many of which I have tried and found helpful. The information about the "zapper" program is derived from the book *The Cure for all Diseases* by Hulda Regehr Clark, Ph.D., N.D.

Dry Brush Technique

The body cleanses itself automatically through eliminative organs such as the kidneys, the liver, the lungs, the lymphatic system, and the skin (the largest one). The accumulation of toxic waste products in body tissues interferes with the nourishment and oxygenation of the cells, leading to degenerative disease and premature aging. Dry skin brushing helps distribution of fat deposits, refresh the complexion, move the lymph, relieve stress, reduce tension, remove dead skin, revitalize the skin, remove skin impurities, keep the pores open, stimulate and increase blood circulation, stimulate hormones, tone the skin, revitalize oil-producing glands, and stimulate nerve endings in the skin. It is best done with a natural bristle brush with a long handle. Start from the head, hands, or feet, and always brush towards the heart.

Ear Wax Candles or Cones

If you have trouble with wax build up in your ears, earwax candles are a solution. You can purchase them at most health food stores for a few dollars. They are very easy to use. They are made of a fine natural cotton or gauze that has been wrapped around a rod and dipped in wax. For convenience and safety, make sure you have someone to help you. A paper plate is also recommended. Make a small hole through the center of the plate. The smaller end of the candle is pushed about four inches through the hole. The patient then lays his or her head horizontally, with the ear to be cleared pointing upward. The small end of the cone is placed in the ear opening (like sticking your finger in your ear). With the paper plate acting as a shield to prevent sparks or ashes from falling onto the hair, the other person lights the candle at the top. The candle is hollow and as the top burns, it warms the earwax. The burning of the top part of the candle absorbs the oxygen in the ear and creates a gentle suction effect that draws the wax from the ear into the hollow opening in the candle. Once the candle burns down to a few inches from the plate, it should be removed and placed in water to douse the burning candle. This process takes six to eight minutes. You can feel heat and hear the sizzle of the candle. Also, you can feel the wax being drawn out. If you are curious about the amount of wax removed, you can cut open the candle to view the brown wax that has collected into the previously hollow center of the candle. Again, do not try doing this by yourself. I use this process about once every eighteen months.

Homeopathic and Holistic Medicine

Homeopathic medicine is based on the "law of similar." It is usually free of side effects, non-toxic, and can be used in combination with regular mainstream treatments. Some of today's pharmaceutical companies are researching homeopathic medicines and natural combinations.

Holistic medicine focuses on the attainment of emotional, mental, physical, social, and spiritual aspects of health. This includes treatment with drugs and surgery if no safe alternative exists.

I have had exposure to the holistic type of medicine. Having an upset stomach has been a very common occurrence for me and was thought to be one of the side effects of my MS. Recently, while getting ready for an alternative treatment at a clinic for homeopathic and nutritional medicine, I told the nurse I had an upset stomach. She offered me a tablet to settle my stomach, and I accepted. Within twenty minutes my stomachache was gone. The tablet I took is called "stomach," and its use is for dyspepsia, heartburn, indigestion, nausea, and stomach discomfort.

KI

KI is a Japanese form of energy healing whereby the technician uses his or her energy to arouse stimuli in a person's body and promote healing. The basis for KI is the natural flow of energy through the body. Each hand has a charge, with the right hand being positive and the left being negative. Placing the hands on parts of the body creates electron movement through the circuit created by the hands. This procedure is usually very quick and pain free. It has been used for many years.

Liver Cleansing

This mixture is to be used on a ten-day fast to help purify the liver. Mix two tablespoons lemon or lime juice, one tablespoon pure grade maple syrup, 1/10 teaspoon cayenne pepper to taste and twelve ounces of purified warm water.

This helps dissolve toxins and cleanse the kidneys and digestive system. It helps purify the glands and cells, eliminate unusable waste and hardened material in joints and muscles, clear congestion, and build a healthy blood system. It also helps relieve irritation and pressure in the nerves, arteries, and blood vessels.

Oxygen Therapy

A finger clip sensor can measure oxygen saturation in the body. This gauges the volume of oxygen in the blood, but not if the oxygen is being transferred to the cells correctly. The oxygen pressure is what is important. Multi-step oxygen therapy improves pressure and carries with it many benefits.

Multi-step oxygen therapy is an eighteen-day exercise program of physical exertion for two hours each day while breathing oxygen at six liters per minute. For every twenty-minute period of exercise, the exertion level should be increased for two minutes. A professional should supervise this program, and after being trained, a person can continue this therapy in his or her own home. There are some precautions to be taken, and the quality of the oxygen is important. The eighteen-day duration can be varied to meet personal need.

Prolotherapy

This is a non-surgical treatment for chronic pain relief. It involves injecting an irritant into the area of pain, which attracts immune cells to the area to rebuild collagen tissue. This causes a healing process with ligaments and tendons that takes pain and pressure off the sensitive nerve or muscle. It could take a couple of treatments to eliminate the pain.

This treatment has been around for fifty years and is very helpful for arthritis, back pain, migraines, sciatica, sports injuries, tendonitis, and TMJ (Temporomandibular Joint Syndrome).

Reflexology

Reflexology is an art all to itself. Your body has nerve endings in your hands and feet that a trained reflexologist can manipulate and energize to create balance and force out toxins. It promotes healing by applying pressure on various reflex points to relieve symptoms elsewhere in the body.

The feet contain twenty acupoints that have connections through the body. All of the organs in the body show up in the chart that the reflexologist uses. The use of heat can enhance the process.

Reflexology is primarily massaging the feet but can also be done to the hands, lower legs, or back. It is not a diagnostic tool even though problem areas can be noted during treatment. After starting with a gentle foot massage, the reflexologist applies pressure to reflex points corresponding to your health problems. The toes correspond to the head and neck, the ball of the foot to the chest and lungs, the arch to the internal organs, and the heel to the sciatic nerve and pelvic area. A powder or lotion may be used to make manipulation easier.

Reflexology can help relieve a wide variety of stress-related problems such as: arthritis, asthma, digestive disorders, headaches, irritable bowel syndrome, premenstrual syndrome, sciatica, skin conditions, and even some neurological symptoms like those seen in multiple sclerosis. Self-administered reflexology techniques can be learned from a practitioner.

Reflexology has been around for many years as noted by ancient scrolls. The Chinese, Japanese, and Indian people all worked with their feet to combat illness. The effect is similar to acupuncture but not to be confused with it.

Some reflexologists believe that manipulation of the feet reduces the amount of lactic acid in the tissues while releasing tiny calcium crystals accumulated in nerve endings that hold back the flow of energy to corresponding organs. Other practitioners believe that pressure on reflex points may trigger the release of chemicals in the brain that naturally block pain, and others believe the therapy opens blood vessels and improves circulation. While none of this has been scientifically proven, a number of people have experienced benefits from the more than twenty-five thousand practitioners worldwide.

Persons with foot injuries, blood clots, thrombosis, phlebitic ulcers, or other vascular problems should discuss reflexology with their doctors first before doing treatments. Persons with pacemakers, gallstones, kidney stones, or who are pregnant should tell the reflexologist before treatment. Other than these precautionary measures, there are no known side effects. Reflexology is not a substitute for regular medical care. (Some reflexology charts are shown in the appendix.)

Reiki

This is a very old form of eastern healing. Reiki written in Japanese is "Rei-ki." The "rei" means spirit, and "ki" means life force energy. This type of treatment is similar to KI and is a form of energy healing. It is relaxing and works with the mind, body, and spirit. The treatment, prior to an operation, can help promote healing.

Reiki helps to relieve anxiety and stress by balancing energy inside the body. Bad energy and blockages can be altered or removed through proper techniques and practice.

Reiki is done with the hands by touch or passing them over the body. There are seven "trigger points" called chakras on the body; these chakras relate to different parts of the body or body functions. Immediate benefits can sometimes be recognized, and the heat from the energy is usually apparent during treatment. After experiencing treatment, the force of the energy can be sensed with certain techniques. It can be self administered after being taught.

I recently had this done for the first time. Some slight benefit was noticed. Energy was better, and the tingling sensation in my arms eased.

A chart of chakras can be found in the appendix.

Zapper Program

Hulda Regelr Clark puts forth the premise that all diseases are caused by parasites and pollutants. By killing the bacteria, fungi, parasites, viruses, removing the toxins, and supplementing with herbs and food factors, the body can heal itself.

The "Auto-Zap" is a frequency generator (434 KHz–421 KHz) that kills fluke parasites. If you stop re-infecting yourself, along with this program, healing will begin. Use at least once a week, but daily use is safe and more beneficial.

The following seven-step program will get you started.

A Program for Better Health

- Give up red meat. It is okay to eat chicken, turkey, and fish.
- Give up dairy products. Use rice milk (vanilla flavored with vitamin C, D, & calcium is good) on cereals.
- Give up sugar. Eat no candies, sweets, or white sugar. Using stevia is okay.
- Give up alcohol. Drink no beer, wines, or liquor.
- Buy a zapper at your local health food store or online. My recommendation is to use it at least once a week.

- Read the book *The Cure for all Diseases* by Hulda Clark, which explains the theory behind the zapper and other helpful information.

This is a low cost thing to do. You should start to notice improvements in a few days. How long you continue is up to you, but once you stop the healing process, you can fall back to your previous habits. It takes will power. Good luck!

CHAPTER 12
Alternative Testing Methods

This chapter outlines different methods of investigating illness. The information on kinesiology and muscle testing in this chapter came from my own research and experiences.

Background

Normally when you get sick, you go to the doctor to find out what is wrong. After an exam, the doctor might give you a shot and write one or two prescriptions. Does this sound familiar? The doctor almost always treats the symptoms and does not search for what caused the problems. Sometimes the doctor will offer advice on how to prevent the symptoms from happening again.

You are the captain of your own ship (your body), so be knowledgeable about what is going on. If eating something makes you sick, stop eating it. That sounds simple. If you do not know what is making you sick, try to find out. You may not be able to completely reverse a condition, but there are some ways to help manage it. First, you have to find out what is causing the problems. The following pages offer some suggestions that may help.

Bilateral Carotid Doppler Test

This is a simple test to determine blood flow properties in different parts of the body. A gel is applied to certain areas to allow the smooth movement of a tool that monitors the blood flow under the skin. The technician views a monitor and recordings are made. They are looking for hemodynamically significant stenosis or disease, based on segmental systolic pressures, analog waveforms, and pulse volume stenosis in the arteries that are being measured.

Electrodermal Screening

Electrodermal Screening (EDS) is safe and inexpensive. By taking measurements on the skin at certain spots, called meridians, the energy and balance of body systems can be tested. This is based on the traditional Chinese principles of bioenergy (chi), which is the theory behind acupuncture. All internal organs and functions have related channels near the skin surface and can be measured and manipulated by these acupuncture points.

An Electrodermal Screening Device (EDSD) can measure resistance and polarization. This machine has an ohmmeter, a testing probe, a metal plate, and a hand held electrode. The system is connected to a monitor and the results are printed. Pressure applied by the probe is firm and somewhat uncomfortable but not painful. There are approximately 850 measurement points on the body and about forty meridians on the hands and feet. If one part of the body is out of balance, other parts are affected. Reagents or supplements can be set on the metal plate, which will indicate balance or imbalance and can also indicate quantity. This is a test to indicate whether a medicine, herb, or homeopathic remedy is necessary.

Disease is caused by a lack of balance, causing abnormal function to a part of the body. The combination of mainstream medical science and EDS has not really been used to any great extent.

Some of my EDS results are shown in the appendix.

Electron Beam Angiography

Computed Tomography Imaging (CT Scan, CAT Scan) was developed in the 1970s. This is a relatively new, fast, safe, and non-invasive procedure using electron beam computed tomography that can give ten to twenty years of advanced warning for some of the most serious diseases. Centers that do this are popping up all over the country. The FDA has given market clearance for Electron Beam Angiography (EBA).

These full body CAT scan x-rays provide 3-D imaging of the inside of a person's body. The computer software technology allows a licensed radiologist to take a virtual tour from the CD-ROM. This computer program allows rotation and in-depth, organ-by-organ review. Approximately fifty centers and fifteen thousand scans have been completed prior to January of 2003.

Insurance companies do not usually cover these elective procedures, but some are beginning to. The cost is six hundred to a thousand dollars. Actual tests take fifteen minutes plus an hour of review by a radiologist. A patient is required to drink a barium-laced drink, have electrodes attached to the chest, and lay flat on his or her back on a table, fully clothed. The patient is then rolled into the CT scanner machine, similar to a Magnetic Resonance Imaging machine (MRI).

This procedure can give early detection of potential diseases such as breast, colon, and lung cancer. It is very effective in showing cysts, plaque, and polyps. It measures bone mineral density, so it is effective in early detection of osteoporosis. This is a risk management tool and can motivate behavior modifications. Rather than exploratory or unnecessary surgery, this is quick and worth the cost. Sixty-two percent of women who died from heart attacks had no previous warning. This, like other tests, is not 100 percent effective and other tests may be required.

Hair-Mineral Analysis

A hair-mineral analysis is inexpensive, and insurance might cover it. Your hair tells much about what is in your body. When advanced procedures are used, the results are accurate and reliable. Over two hundred thousand of these tests are done each year. The amount of hair necessary to perform this test is small—usually about the amount the barber takes off. It gives your health practitioner direction on where you may need help. It will tell how much aluminum, arsenic, and mercury, along with other not so toxic minerals, are in your body. This is a test you can have repeated after you have been working on corrective measures for a while to see the results of treatments.

Examples of results of my hair-mineral analysis are in the appendix.

Iridology

The science of iridology examines the eyes. It pays little attention to symptoms and deals with prevention. Careful attention must adhere to detailed and perceptive observations. In order to master the concept of iridology, time, dedication, and training are essential.

The anatomy of typical and abnormal conditions is well documented. Iridology cannot determine a disease, but recognizes biochemical deficiencies, general health level, inflammation stages, strength, toxin locations, and weakness. When there is a disorder in the digestive and intestinal tracts, it can be observed in the iris of the eyes, as can the healing progress.

Many medical history factors can be noted in the fibers of the eyes. One of my past experiences with iridology was when my mother thought she'd had a stroke. After a trip to the iridology practitioner, the conclusion was that it could have been a low blood sugar level instead. The iridologist showed us pictures of the eyes of a person who had a stroke. There was a big difference: my mom's eyes were cloudy, but the stroke victim's eyes looked like rays of lightning, all jagged and broken.

Kinesiology

Definition

Kinesiology is the science of muscle testing (MT) to determine energy flow. Allergists, chiropractors, herbalists, laymen, nutritionists, veterinarians, and some doctors use it. MT is part of a relatively new medical field called bioenergetics. MT tests for electrical blockages using an outside stimulator. It is not a test of strength, but measures electrical impulses or oscillations. MT is a simple way of evaluating the electrical circuits of the body through acupuncture points, meridians, or muscles. These meridians run throughout the body just under the skin. The skin is the largest organ in the body and has the same kind of sensors found in the brain. Approximately seventy-five known reflex areas on the skin relate to organs, glands, and bone structure.

Muscle testing is a diagnostic tool if used properly by a trained practitioner. The thymus gland is at the center of the chest, and it influences muscle testing. If the thymus is weak, muscle testing is difficult.

Methods of Testing

There are different types of MT, and overall, it is usually met with criticism. One method of muscle testing is conducted by a person extending his or her arm to the side horizontally, and the practitioner applying pressure to the wrist area to see how much resistance the person can tolerate. Next, the person is asked to hold a product or foodstuff in the other hand against the chest, and pressure is once again applied to the wrist. If the strength is equal, the item is considered beneficial; but if there is a decrease in strength, then it is to be considered detrimental. White cane sugar is not good for you, and by doing a test, there is much difficulty experienced in holding your arm out horizontal.

Another method of this type of testing is done by forming a loop with the index finger and the thumb on one hand and interlocking it with the same loop on the other hand, noting the pressure required to disengage the lock while pulling your arms outward. The product or item you are testing should be in contact with your body, though some practitioners say all you need to do is concentrate on it. I have had muscle testing done to me with some visual effects.

Limitations

The accuracy of MT is qualified by the mind of the person utilizing it. MT does not work when the electrical circuitry of the body is weak. Drinking a glass of water may help electrical impulses and increase the capabilities of MT.

Many people misuse MT, and so respecting kinesiology can be difficult. It is necessary to accept intuition and the field of electromagnetics. A person must learn to feel more and think less. Many people have a hard time accepting something that cannot be identified with the five senses. The 8 percent of the brain we use is controlled by the five senses. The skin should be called our sixth sense.

Keep muscle testing as physiological as possible. You must be neutral and confident in order to be accurate. Predetermined ideas will override testing results and are the key to errors. Requirements for accurate testing are confidence and an indifferent state of mind. In order for any of this to be effective, it is important to believe. Negative thoughts or words will make a muscle test weak.

Simply bringing an item into your body's electromagnetic field can cause blockage. If the item makes your arm go weak simply by holding it, imagine what it does when you ingest it. When an object or food is placed where any of our five senses can detect it, the body will reject it if it is not compatible. If the body senses the item to be positive, the muscle will be strong.

Products with metal encasing should not be tested, but glass and plastic are okay.

Basic Facts

Electricity is the foundation of life. It is proven that the body is electrical when you scuff your feet on a carpet and receive the ensuing shock. Some say your brain can actually connect with someone else's just by thinking of the other person. Sensing that someone is watching you is an example of this theory. By praying for someone, I believe you are actually connecting to him or her on a vibrational level.

Everything in life and on Earth has it's own electromagnetic vibration or energy frequency and can be measured by machines. A few machines have been developed to test electrical deficiencies such as: Electroacupuncture (EAV: $12,000-20,000), Quantum Xrroid Consciousness Interface (QXCI: $13,000), and Scientific Consciousness Operations System (SCIO: $18,000). These machines have been proven to be quite accurate.

Minerals flow in and out of a cell causing the cell to spin in circles and create a vibration. These vibrations flow through organized pathways called meridians. There is an external point on the body that is related through these meridians to every internal part of the body. Every cell in our body contains energy, and we receive bioenergy from everything in our environment. Energy is created in the body, and every cell generates electricity. With a magnet you can feel the field of energy as positive and negative energies are drawn together, but you cannot see it. Magnetic fields indicate that opposites attract.

There are four ways in which energy flows: clockwise (positive), counter-clockwise (negative), vertical (neutral), and oscillating (pulsating). All disease begins with oscillations.

There are two basic nervous systems. The first is voluntary, which the mind controls. The second is autonomic (involuntary), which controls organs and their functions.

Nerves maintain your balance and regulate your body temperature (98.6°F is normal). A complete nerve system is made up of an organ, part of the skin, and a muscle. If nerve energy is flowing freely, the muscle will remain strong. Weakness indicates that nerve energy has been interrupted. When there is any abnormality in the body, the electricity that once flowed through that area is no longer able to flow freely. An Electrocardiogram (EKG) test works on the same principle of electrical impulses.

Thermology

Thermology is the study of heat. With the use of an infrared thermal imaging machine, a map of the body can be assessed. Long ago, the Greeks and Egyptians used their hands and fingers to sense heat and cold to monitor disease. Galileo developed a thermoscope to measure body temperature. It was Fahrenheit and Wunderlich who established the thermometer as we know today, yet all the early methods were contact methods.

In the last thirty years, infrared thermal imaging methods have been developed and are highly sensitive, emitting degrees of colors to note the spectrum of heat found. This procedure can be beneficial in the diagnosis and treatment of carpal tunnel syndrome, poor circulation, muscles tears, forearm myopathy, neuro-vascular activity, thermographic abnormalities, symptomatology, and vibration sensitivity. The scans are done while laying on a platform fully dressed, minus shoes and accessories.

There are not many facilities that do thermology, so it may take some digging to locate one. My tests showed marked regions of poor circulation more pronounced in my left leg, causing poor function. It also showed the Basal Cell Carcinoma on my forehead. (Printouts of my tests are shown in the appendix.)

CHAPTER 13
Cancer, Colon, and Yeast

Much of the information in this chapter about cancer was derived from the monthly newsletter *Health and Healing* by Julian Whitaker, M.D. Much of the information about yeast was derived from the book *The Yeast Connection* by William G. Crook, M.D.

Cancer

Definition

Cancer is caused by the uncontrollable division of body cells. When this happens, a malignant tumor is formed that enlarges and may spread. Cancer is tenacious—sometimes subsiding, but reappearing years later after a presumed cure. Cells from the primary tumor can break off, lodge elsewhere, and grow into secondary tumors. This process is called metastasis.

In America, one out of three will get cancer, and one out of five will die from it. Cancer claims the lives of about fifteen hundred people per day. The average person's chance of acquiring cancer in 1960 was one in four. In 1994, this rose to two in five. Much research is being done using gene and stem cell therapy.

Diagnosis

Being diagnosed with cancer is a process that does not happen all at once. Until a pathologist has examined a sample of the tumor from a biopsy, the exact type of cancer may not be known. Appropriate treatment depends on things such as location, type, appearance, and size.

Types

Types of cancer include: bone, brain, breast, cervical, colorectal, endocrine system, gastrointestinal, head, Hodgkin' disease, kidney, leukemia, lung, lymphomas, metastases, myelomas, Non-Hodgkin's lymphoma, oral, ovarian, pediatric, penile, prostate, sarcomas, skin, testicular, thyroid, urinary tract, and uterine.

Mammography, involving a low intensity x-ray of the breast, is the most common form of breast cancer testing. The breasts have to be flattened to get the best picture. There are mixed opinions by professionals as to the accuracy of this procedure. There is another method that is more accurate without the radiation and flattening. It is called infrared thermography. It measures heat sensitivity emitted by new cell growth, a process called neoangiogenesis. This process is over 90 percent effective, as opposed to 65 to 80 percent for mammography. Its ability to detect small tumors is much greater. For those persons interested, log onto www.breastthermography.com.

The possibility of prostate cancer could be reduced by nearly 60 percent with the use of 200 mcg per day of yeast-derived selenium, as it is a powerful antioxidant. A study also found the incidence of prostate cancer reduced by 40 percent in men with high levels of Omega-3 fish oils in their blood.

Most skin cancers are caused by Basel cells and show up on the ears, head, and neck. An alternative to surgery is to try a paste of Dimethyl Sulfoxide (DMSO), shark cartilage, and vitamin C powder applied to the spot a couple times a day.

Causes

Some of the most recognized causes of cancer are viruses, chemical carcinogens, environmental hazards, heredity, nutrition, and radiation.

Possible indications or warnings are: changes in bowel or bladder habits, sores, that do not heal, unusual bleeding or discharge, lumps in the skin, indigestion or difficulty in swallowing, an obvious change in a mole or wart, and a nagging cough or hoarseness.

The National Cancer Institute found that farmers exposed to pesticides and herbicides have a three to six times greater chance of contracting certain types of cancer.

Labeling

A Roman numeral usually indicates the stage of cancer, with IV being the most severely progressed. Another way of labeling cancer is the TNM method (T = tumor, N = lymph nodes and M = metastasis). A T1N1M0 represents a tumor from T0 through T4, regional lymph from N1 through N4, and metastasis from M1 through M2.

Treatments

Conventional treatments are surgery (cutting out the cancer), chemotherapy (poisoning the cells), and radiation (burning the cells). Their rate of success is not always very good. Insurance companies will pay for the conventional treatments but will not if you go the alternative route.

Alternative Treatment 1

Two stories come to mind when I think of cancer. The first is of a nurse in Canada who, through treatment with a Native American concoction, was curing people. The nurse's name was Rene Caisse and her efforts had cured over 450 people. The tea she was brewing for treatment was called Essiac, and it consists of a blend of burdock root, sheep's sorrel, slippery elm, and Indian rhubarb root. Rumor has it, though I could not confirm, that the Canadian government found out about it, raided her house, confiscated her records, and burned them.

The mixture for Essiac tea is still available. Essiac tea is available through a company called "Enrich." Thousands claim to have been cured using Essiac tea. Another company, Nature's Sunshine, has put the same ingredients into a capsule called "E-Tea."

Conventional treatments—chemotherapy, radiation, and surgery—believe you have to kill the cancer cells whereas Essiac tea helps to purify the blood and nourish the cells. It may increase the odds of improvement.

Alternative Treatment 2

The second story relates to a Polish immigrant named Stanislaw Burzynski, M.D., Ph.D. He uses antineoplastons, which are naturally occurring peptides (small protein components) that regulate cell growth. Cancer generally develops from defects in the genes of our cells. The two classes of genes are normally in balance, but they are suppressed in persons with cancer. These are oncogenes, which regulate growth, and tumor suppressor genes, which suppress growth. By developing a process for synthesizing antineoplastons and administering them, cancer cells are not destroyed, but cell growth is normalized. Dr. Burzynski has endured four grand juries, two trials, and a criminal indictment of fifteen charges. He has been vindicated in every instance. A couple of web sites with further information are: cancermed.com and burzynskipatientgroup.org.

Alternative Treatment 3

There is another treatment that has been successful in treating breast, lung, and prostate cancer. It is called Insulin Potentiation Therapy (IPT). It has been around for forty years. A Dr. Perez, who is located in Tijuana, Mexico, uses it. The treatment works on cancer cells and their ability to consume glucose. Cancer cells are dependant on glucose and require insulin. The treatment affects this process, making the cells more exceptive to insulin and also making them more receptive to chemotherapy drugs.

Alternative Treatment 4

Artemisinin is an herbal extract that works like chemotherapy without the side effects. Artemisinin is not a stand-alone chemotherapeutic agent. Artemisinin, when used with Carnivora, CoQ10, green tea, and pancreatic enzyme, was found beneficial. In experiments, it was found to have a high propensity for accumulating iron, which is high in cancer cells.

Alternative Treatment 5

Another treatment that shows promise is in the June 2000 issue of *Second Opinion*. Dr. Rowen discusses resveratrol, a natural anti-fungal agent found in grapes. A product called Resveratrol Plus is available on the market. It is not a stand-alone treatment for cancer and dosages of three to five a day are recommended.

Alternative Treatment 6

The Gerson therapy combines detoxification with nutrition aimed at restoring immunity and the natural healing of the body. Max Gerson found the blood of cancer patients was deficient in certain nutrients that allowed cancer cells to grow out of control. The diet is the core of this therapy, which protects against the development of cancer and helps fight existing cancer.

Alternative Treatment 7

A relatively new form of light therapy for cancer is Cytoluminescent Therapy (CLT). This uses a chemical called a photosensitizer. This chemical absorbs light of a certain wavelength, which generates massive quantities of free radicals that attack cancer cells. Normal cells do not absorb much of this photosensitizing chemical and are not harmed.

Prevention

Cancer prevention is not an exact science. Therapies and healthy living can act as deterrents. Consider these recommendations: avoiding environmental carcinogens and tobacco, eating a healthy diet, exercising, avoiding alcohol, and watching your weight. Protective antioxidants can also reduce your risks. .

Some suggestions for cancer prevention are to start taking hydrazine sulfate and switch to a mostly vegetarian diet. Reduce calorie intake to approximately fifteen hundred at least three times a week. Take aloe vera juice, barley grass juice, CoQ10, either bovine or shark cartilage, micropolysaceharides, pycnogenol, and vitamin C. Certain foods may help in prevention such as: broccoli, brussel sprouts, cabbage, cauliflower, kale, pomegranates, rutabaga, and turnips.

Milk and dairy products have been tested as strong promoters of some types of cancer. Dietary lactose, a sugar found in milk, may increase the risk of ovarian cancer; and for every 11 grams per day, the risk is increased by approximately 19 percent. Dairy products also have a high fat content and environmental toxins.

Broccoli and other brassica vegetables contain sulforaphane that helps destroy the microbe Helicobacter pylori, a possible cause of duodenal ulcers, stomach cancer, and stomach ulcers. Sulforaphane kills germs in the stomach lining.

Colon

Rumor has it that 90 percent of our diseases originate in the colon. Most people are concerned with keeping the outside of their bodies clean and healthy, but the number of people who take reasonable care to keep their insides clean is small. It is difficult to find the necessary discipline for the required processes to do a thorough cleaning. Also, it is not a one-time shot; it should be repeated on a yearly basis. The build up of impacted fetal material on the linings of the intestines is a breeding ground for harmful bacteria, parasites, and toxins. The necessary treatments take time, but you will be surprised by how well you feel just a short time into a program.

Clean and active bowels promote the passing of waste and toxins that can otherwise build up. Regularity differs person to person from three times a week to three times a day. Constipation can be impaction that presses on nerves and can cause abdominal and back pain. Some medicines for blood pressure, cancer, and depression, including antacids, antihistamines, and cough suppressants, can cause constipation. Cramps, fatigue, irregular heartbeat, muscle cramps, and a potassium deficiency are early signs of constipation. Laxatives deplete potassium. Professional medical practitioners recommend that you do not use laxatives if you have kidney problems, as they draw water from surrounding body tissue. Foods rich in potassium such as avocados, bananas, cantaloupe, dried fruits, and leafy greens are rich in potassium and therefore bowel-friendly. Improve general body health and bowel function by drinking plenty of good fluids, eating a healthy diet, and exercising.

Yeast

Definition

Yeast is a single cell fungus, which normally lives in the intestines and other parts of the digestive tract. When yeasts multiply, they emit toxins that weaken the immune system and cause illness. Many things encourage yeast growth. Everyone has a certain amount of yeast in his or her body, and when your immune system is strong, they do not bother you. If you have taken anti-biotics, cortisone, prednisone, or other corticosteroids, chances are you might have acquired a yeast infection. The antibiotics destroy the good bacteria in your intestine and are an invitation for the candidiasis (yeast) to take over. You may not know this has happened. Diets rich in sugar and yeast are also contributors. It can spread to your bloodstream, the ears, the throat, and the vagina. Yeast lowers your immune system's ability to overcome bacteria, fungus, and toxin build up.

Symptoms

Symptoms are acne, allergies, asthma, bloating, bronchitis, congestion, constipation, cramps, depression, exhaustion, fatigue, headaches, hives, lack of coordination, infections, irritability, muscle or joint pain, nervousness, numbness, persistent coughs, poor memory, premenstrual syndrome, psoriasis, rash, skin irritations, vaginitis, and weakness.

Treatment

It is difficult to get rid of yeast. It is imperative when trying to combat a yeast infection that a person adheres very strictly to a yeast destructive diet. This means no alcohol, buttermilk, cakes, candies, cantaloupe, carob, cheeses, coffee, condiments, cookies, corn syrup, dextrose, dried fruits, fructose, honey, hydrogenated oils, ice cream, maple syrup, meat, MSG, mushrooms, mustard, packaged or processed food, pastries, peanuts, pickles, raised breads, salad dressings, sauces, soft drinks, sour cream, spices, sugar, tea, tofu, and vinegar. Avoid all foods that promote yeast growth. Avoid all fruit for the first month.

Eat raw or steamed vegetables, brown rice, chicken, eggs, fish, fresh-made vegetable juices, greens of all kind, high fiber grains, fresh juices, lean beef, lean pork, lamb, turkey, seafood, seeds, sprouts, unprocessed nuts and oils, veal, yogurt (sugar free), water, and whole grains.

Treatment involves acrylic acid, citrus seed extract, garlic, herbs, Nystatin (drug), Pau D'Arco, vitamin A, vitamin C, vitamin E, and chlorophyll. These things replace the destroyed bacteria with lactobacillus and acidophilus. Certain dietary supplements, such as broccoli, cabbage, garlic, onions, turnips, and plain yogurt are effective in the curing process. Rebuild the immune system with nutrients like pantothenic acid and thymus substance.

There are certain medications that help rid the body of yeast germs such as Nystatin or other anti-fungal treatments. Treatment with Nystatin may take up to a year. Also, in severe conditions, Diflucan (fluconazole) is a drug used to treat AIDS, Chronic Fatigue Syndrome, and severe depression of the immune system. Other drugs include Nizoral (ketoconazole) and Sporanox (itraconazole). It is important to be patient with treatment, as yeast problems will not go away immediately. In many cases, it can take many months.

CHAPER 14
Interesting Tidbits

This chapter is full of interesting facts that I have come across in my research. Information in this chapter has come from many sources. Most information resulted from the monthly newsletters Second Opinion *by William Campbell Douglas, M.D., and* Health and Healing *by Julian Whitaker, M.D. Information about SSRIs came from the September 1999 issue of the monthly newsletter* Health and Healing *by Julian Whitaker, M.D.*

Food Related

- Almonds—a handful—every day can help lower your LDL cholesterol.
- Apricots can help your sex drive.
- Carrots can help prevent strokes by eating one a day.
- Celery can help bring your blood pressure down.
- Cherries may help fight cancer.
- Cranberry juice and blueberries have been effective in preventing and fighting urinary tract and bladder infections.
- Garlic helps lower cholesterol and triglycerides, block cancer cell growth, and fight bacterial infections.
- Grapefruits, lemons, limes, and oranges rolled on a counter or between your hands before cutting open will increase the juice output.
- Grapefruit may help prevent breast cancer. Grapefruit and grapefruit juice may have a side effect that prevents the enzymes in the liver from metabolizing certain types of drugs including therapeutic drugs. With drugs of this type, it would be a good idea to check their compatibility. Eat grapefruit or drink the juice in moderation. Red grapefruit is healthier than white.
- Honey can help heal wounds.
- Oysters are well known as an aphrodisiac.
- Rice (brown) soaked overnight in warm water before cooking the next day increases its germination process to release important nutrients.
- Roasted nuts can help prevent heart attacks.
- Tomatoes (cooked) are a source of lycopene, which is linked to a reduced risk of prostate cancer. Drinking a can of low sodium tomato juice instead of soda pop will help lower your risk of heart disease.

- Drinking lots of water is the best way to stop kidney stone formation. Add unsweetened lemon concentrate to help increase the prevention of stones.
- If your fingernails are chipping or breaking, it is a possible indication that your body does not have enough water. Drink more water and soon you should notice stronger nails.
- Yogurt helps digest dairy products and increase the level of interferon, which is an immune enhancing hormone.

Foods Recommended

A list of some foods recommended for better health are as follows: almonds, amaranth flour, apples, applesauce, apricots, bananas (unsweetened), beef (lean), beans (black, navy, and red), bean soup (homemade), blackberries, blueberries, bread (Ezekiel sprouted grains), cashews, cherries, cranberries, dates, fish (cold-water hormone and chemical free), flaxseed oil, garlic, grapes (red), kiwi, lamb, mangos, millet, olive oil (virgin), pears, potatoes (red), rabbit, raisins, raspberries, rice (brown), rice drink, quinoa, sea salt (unprocessed), smelt, soy, veal, vegetable soup (homemade), venison, walnuts, water (oxygenated and purified), and Westsoy vanilla soy.

Foods not Recommended

A list of some of the foods which are not recommended for optimum health are as follows: alcohol, artificial sweeteners, artificial vanilla, A-1 steak sauce, barley, bay leaves, beans (kidney and lima), Brazil nuts, buckwheat, caffeine, canola oil, cinnamon, coconut, condiments made with vinegar, corn, corn beef, corn oil, corn syrups, curry, dairy products, eggs (supermarket), fish (bottom feeders and shellfish), food dyes, garbanzo, grapefruit, hydrogenated oils, lemons, lentils, lunch meats, margarine, meats (smoked), melons (especially during winter), MSG, mushrooms, oats, paprika, peas (split), pecans, peanuts, pepper (black), peppers, pineapple, popcorn, poppy seeds, pistachio nuts, potatoes (white), pumpkin, safflower oil, sage, salt (table), soups (boxed or ready-to-go), soy sauce, strawberries, sunflower seeds, tea (black), tea (with caffeine), vegetable oil, and wheat.

Health Improvement Recommendations

- Beer (dark) and wine in moderate amounts help reduce the risk of heart disease. The benefits of bioflavonoids, found in beer and wine, appear to cease after one drink for women and two drinks for men.

- Caffeine can help increase endurance, as it is a mild stimulant, which increases the breakdown of fat. Benefits are temporary and continued use is detrimental to your overall health.
- Coconut milk is helpful in the preventative to Montezuma's revenge.
- Creatine monohydrate is a natural supplement and using up to 5 grams per day Alternative Testing Methodshelps build larger muscles. Side effects can be abdominal cramping and water retention.
- Exercise (resistance), once a week, can help improve muscle strength in older adults.
- Headaches may be eased by the massage of the meaty part of your hand between your thumb and index finger.
- Healing wounds can best be accomplished by gently washing the wound with soap and water and then applying some zinc oxide. Sugar helps fights bacterial growth by drawing fluids out of the wound. Apply a sterile covering to the area to maintain a moist environment. The idea of leaving a wound exposed to air for healing is incorrect.
- Heartburn and indigestion can be improved by drinking warm water with a teaspoon of organic apple cider vinegar and a little bit of honey if desired.
- Hiccups might disappear if you massage your ear lobes.
- High homocysteine levels can be reduced by vitamins B6, B12, and folic acid.
- Neural therapy is effective in treating joint pain when only one joint is affected. It involves the use of Procaine injections. Scar therapy is very similar.
- Potassium-magnesium aspartate is helpful as an endurance booster.
- Six facets of not having optimum health are: no exercise, genetics, malnutrition, physical impairment, stress, and toxins. Genetic health problems are the most difficult to change because you are born with them. This might affect how well your body is able to metabolize certain vitamins.
- Rubbing the site of a mosquito or bee sting with a cut onion helps ease itching.
- The recommended steak serving size by the USDA is only 3 ounces where as the average American restaurant serving is 12 ounces.
- Testosterone is a hormone in both men and women related to sexual desire. Low levels can be treated with dehydroepiandrosterone (DHEA) sold in health food stores. It is a good idea to start with low inputs of 25 mg per day or less.

- The Law of Herring states that healing must take place from top to bottom, inside out, and in reverse order.
- Weight loss is a concern for many people. To help with weight loss it is a good idea to increase both your calcium and vitamin C input. A calcium deficiency causes the body to store fat. Overweight individuals might want to consider having a glucose tolerance test. These tests find out the body's ability to handle carbohydrates and insulin. High levels of insulin raise homocysteine levels, which lead to vascular disease and diabetes. Hunger is a sign your body needs something. Eat when you are hungry and stop when the craving is satisfied. You don't have to eat just because it is mealtime.
- The average life span is 74.9 years. As a person ages, the digestive system brakes down and our bodies produce fewer enzymes and hormones, which affect the endocrine system. These enzymes are secreted in the adrenals, the hypothalamus, the ovaries, the pancreas, the pineal, the pituitary, the testes, the thymus, and the thyroid. As we age the secretion of hydrochloric acid and pepsin decreases, impairing digestion along with reduced absorption of biotin, calcium, iron, and vitamin B12.
- Natural hormone replacement is generally safer than prescriptions. To help keep your stomach healthy, supplements of delycyrrhizinayed (DGL), licorice, papain, and bromelain can help. Most of the digestion process is done in the small intestine. As digestion decreases, constipation, cramping, diverticulosis, lower stomach pain, and ulcers can occur.
- Avoid bathing or showering during a thunderstorm as the plumbing can conduct electricity from lightning.
- Constipation may be helped by chewing your food thoroughly, drinking lots of water, cutting back on the input of alcohol, aspirins, caffeine, and NSAIDS. Also try adding flaxseed to your diet.
- To help discourage the craving for alcohol, take a lot of vitamins and minerals. Alcoholism is a disease that is related to inadequate intake of nutrients.
- Eating a lot of hot dogs and other processed meat doubles the risk of colon cancer and type II diabetes.
- Iron is a valuable mineral in the body, as it is necessary for the red blood cells to transport oxygen. Deficiency can cause abdominal pain, angina, fatigue, heart palpitations, impotence, and joint pain. Excess iron can also cause problems such as constipation, a flush face, and high blood pressure. There is

no natural way for the body to rid itself of excess iron. Chelation can help reduce levels of iron that can be detected using a ferritin-level test.

- Macular degeneration (age-related) prevention can be helped and some deterioration reversed by eating certain foods that are low in fat and high in nutrients (carotenoids) and strengthen the eyes. Antioxidants in fruits and vegetables (orange and dark green), whole grains, and legumes can help show eye improvement. Taking supplements like CoQ10, Omega-3, selenium, and zinc, and a diet rich in lutein also will help.

- Low levels of magnesium could be the cause of low energy.

- Mercury poisoning is a serious health risk. Symptoms can take years to develop. Mercury amalgam fillings release vapor when you chew food, brush or grind your teeth, or drink hot beverages. Some fish have high mercury content, mainly bigger fish. The risk of heart disease is increased with high levels of mercury. Mercury in the body crosses the blood-brain barrier easily and attacks the brain and nervous system along with reducing the activity of immune cells. Symptoms of mercury poisoning include numbness, tingling, loss of coordination, tremors, fatigue, weakness, dizziness, headaches, memory loss, depression, and irritability. A hair evaluation will tell the mercury content in your body. The DMPS challenge is also a test for mercury levels in the body. Administering DMPS, a chelating compound, by IV or injection will attach to some of the mercury and allow the body to pass it off as waste. After the DMPS therapy, measuring the amount of mercury in the urine calculates the amount of mercury stored in the body. A drug called Chemet can be used also.

- To cut down on mosquitoes bothering you, try putting a couple drops of Lemon Joy dishwashing soap on a white plate with water in it nearby. The mosquitoes will be attracted to the plate and ingestion of the soap will kill them.

- Stress helps reduce the body's ability to fight infection and increase stomach-acid levels. It can also cause aging and wrinkles.

- A dead or missing tooth or root canal can be traumatic and irritate the nervous system.

- Ulcers can be caused by infection.

- Ultraviolet radiation (UVA) from a tanning booth is approximately 2.5 times more damaging to the skin than direct sunlight.

- Viagra diminishes an enzyme in the body that restricts nitric oxide. Nitric oxide is necessary for dilation of blood vessels and increases blood flow in the penis. Side effects are that it is highly reactive and toxic, and increased blood flow in the brain and eyes can lead to free radical damage.

A Good Night's Sleep

- We usually do not pay enough attention to sleep. After all, we spend approximately a third of our lives sleeping. How we sleep dictates how we function during the other two thirds of our lives. Emotional, environmental, or physical things can disturb good sleep.

- There are three kinds of sleep: light sleep, deep sleep, and dream sleep. Light sleep happens when we first drop off. Deep sleep happens when our bodies are in a completely relaxed state and usually only lasts for intervals, maybe up to ninety minutes. Dream sleep or rapid eye movement (REM) happens when we wake or first go to bed, our muscles are active, and our brain is in gear. Our breathing becomes erratic and vivid dreams or nightmares become apparent.

- As we age, we tend to go to bed earlier and get up earlier with more arousals during sleep. There are many common sleep disorders, including apnea, cataplexy, insomnia, narcolepsy, parasomnia, restless leg syndrome, sleep paralysis, and somnambulism (sleep walking).

- Good sleep hygiene can help to get a good night's sleep. This involves being comfortable in a quiet bed and going to bed at approximately the same time each night. Do not exercise just prior to bed or drink a lot of fluids. Alcohol, drugs, and tobacco can influence sleep.

- If you are having trouble going to sleep, after twenty minutes of sleeplessness, get up and go to another room for some quiet time (not TV). Return to bed when sleepiness is felt. There are many drugs on the market to help with sleep and they should be carefully evaluated before use as they can be habit forming, and may be detrimental to your overall health.

- Snoring is a symptom of sleep apnea, periods of breathing cessation, and REM. There is treatment called continuous positive airway pressure (CPAP). This is a respiratory therapy used to force air into the nasal passage and lungs. Persons with sleep apnea, pulmonary edema, and respiratory distress syndrome can use a CPAP machine.

Medical Facts

- Allergies are one of the most under-accessed causes of body disorders. Most common allergens are found in eggs, fish, milk, peanuts, shellfish, soy, and wheat.
- Alzheimer's disease is diagnosed at the rate of approximately 375,000 patients per year. It causes dementia, mental deterioration, memory loss, and physical characteristic changes. There is a compound on the market called galantamine, which is an ingredient in certain supplements. It can be found at health food stores and will help with dementia. It is a good idea to start with a low dose, 8 mg per day or less. A high input of vitamin C and vitamin E will help reduce the risk of this disease. Taking curcumin can also help slow the effects. Aluminum is suspected of causing Alzheimer's, so drinking from aluminum cans will add minute traces to your body.
- Antibiotics lower the immune response and doctors tend to over-prescribe them. Antibiotics work for treating bacterial infections but do not work for viral infections.
- Arthritis affects eight out of ten persons by age fifty-five. Conventional medicine treats arthritis with non-steroidal anti-inflammatory drugs (NSAIDs) such as Celebrex and Vioxx. Long-term use of this type of drug has been linked to about one hundred thousand hospitalizations and sixteen thousand deaths every year. Side effects include bleeding, damage to gastrointestinal tract, nausea, stomach upset, and ulcers. These drugs can cause a reaction when taken with alcohol, blood thinners, diuretics, Fluconazole, lithium, methotrexate, and steroids. Natural oral supplements are Methylsulfonylmethane (MSM), Glucosamine, and chondroitin sulfate, which help relieve inflammation, pain, and stiffness, and act as water-holding agents. These supplements affect proteoglycans and macromolecules in the body that help supply nutrients and protect cartilage. They work slowly but are safe if intelligently used.
- Chronic use of NSAIDs for pain increases the risk of GI and kidney and liver damage. Some herbal remedies such as bromelain, curcumin, feverfew, and white willow could offer alternative help.
- There are more than two million adverse drug reactions each year resulting in over one hundred thousand deaths. Drugs are strong chemical agents with many side effects, toxicities, and reactions. Almost all drugs are chemicals and

toxic. Millions of patients each year have reactions to prescription drugs severe enough to cause permanent disability or hospitalization. "One dose fits all" is not true.

- Hypertension is a condition of high blood pressure. It can cause Alzheimer's, dementia, diabetes, heart failure, kidney problems, and strokes if not dealt with. Mainstream doctors treat hypertension with drugs that are toxic and have many side effects. A baby aspirin at bedtime can help reduce blood pressure. Natural approaches to treatment are slower but safer. To help with this problem, avoid excess alcohol, cut back on salt, exercise, lose weight, stop smoking, and eat a healthy diet. Eat more fruits and vegetables to help increase your potassium.

- Insulin resistance is the body's way of blocking glucose and other nutrients from getting into the cells. This causes blood sugar to rise and increases body fat. Refined carbohydrates, sugar, and white flour are all contributors to insulin resistance and cutting back on bread, high-starch foods, pastries, white potatoes, and white rice will help.

- Leaky Gut Syndrome (LGS) is a condition where the intestines develop larger than normal holes that allow allergens and infectious pathogens to enter the body. Food allergies pass into the system this way, and the immune system releases chemical antibodies, such as histamine or seratonin, in an effort to protect the body. The cause for LGS can be alcohol, antibiotics, birth control pills, coffee, soda pop, or steroids.

- Lyme's disease may be helped through use of a zapper.

- Prescription drugs kill up to two hundred thousand people a year, making them the third largest cause of death, right behind cancer and heart disease.

- The drug Ritalin is sometimes misused. It is used to treat children with attention deficit hyperactivity disorder (ADHD). Side effects of this amphetamine-like drug are agitation, loss of appetite, stunted growth, and upset stomach.

- Selective serotonin reuptake inhibitors (SSRIs) are a popular form of antidepressants such as Effexor, Luvox, Paxil, Prozac, and Zoloft. These are prescription drugs that can be dangerous. These drugs can trigger violent and suicidal behavior. They increase the level of serotonin in the brain. Prescribed as treatment for depression, these drugs are mind altering. They cause a condition called akathisia. They can cause serious side effects such as aggression, agitation, anxiety, emotional detachment, depression, headache, loss of libido, nausea, nervousness, paranoia, poor appetite, restlessness, sleep disorder, suicidal thoughts, and violence. In one out of twenty-five children it causes exalted feelings, delusions of grandeur, and wild ideas. It causes a dissociative reaction, so logic and reason are impaired. One out of twelve patients admitted to mental hospitals for psychosis take SSRIs. If you are presently taking an SSRI and plan on stopping, it is dangerous to do it instantly. Some milder and safer antidepressants are S-adenosyl-methionine (SAMe), St. John's wort, and 5-hydroxytryprophan (5-HTP).

- Statin drugs are commonly used to treat high cholesterol. As an alternative, the combination of red yeast extract, CoQ10, and guggul is also effective. Red yeast extract contains natural phytochemicals including mevinolin, which is one of the compounds found in lovastatin, and is a compound in nature. Red yeast extract is natural and should be started with a low dose under the watchful eye of a health practitioner.

- Symptoms of under-active thyroid are chronic infections, cold hands and feet, constipation, depression, fatigue, headaches, high cholesterol, infertility, memory difficulties, menstrual irregularities, skin and hair problems, slow heartbeat, slow wound healing, and weight gain. Natural thyroid replacement supplements are available like garlic, niacin, and other lipid-lowering agents. A routine blood test, called the thyrotropin test, measures the thyroid's activity.

- Try to avoid the intake of toxins if possible. Eat organic foods and avoid drugs (big toxic threat), smoke, and chemical inhalation. Do not allow your dentist to use mercury.

- The drug Xanax, used for nerves, is more addictive than Valium and may cause rage and hostility.

Supplement Facts

- It is very helpful to take acidolophis in large doses when taking antibiotics to put good flora back into your stomach. The antibiotics may cause stomach pains. Bacterial colitis is the medical term used when, after taking antibiotics, you have destroyed the good bacteria in your stomach. Bad bacteria replace the pockets of good bacteria.

- If you want a boost of energy, try putting a squirt of liquid aminos in a glass of water in the morning and again at lunchtime. Your body does not produce all the aminos it needs. Amino acids are the building blocks of the human body.

- L-carnosine has anti-aging properties and helps the skin.
- Chaparral may help to reduce the size of cancer tumors.
- Children should take a multivitamin daily.
- Codeine and Demerol are quite helpful for migraine headaches
- Docosahexaenoic acid (DHA) is important in brain function and helps improve circulation by preventing platelets from sticking together. It is a good idea to take two fish oil supplements with eiosapentaenoic acid (EPA) and DHA with meals daily.
- Minerals such as zinc and selenium help strengthen the immune system and ward off viral infections. To treat cold sores, apply ice for ten minutes every hour and use a supplement of L-Lysine.
- To treat the common cold and flu, the use of goldenseal, echinacea, and extra vitamin C as immune boosters can be helpful. Be careful when using goldenseal as it may be allergenic to some people and serious side effects can occur. These supplements should not be taken for periods longer than seven days without a break.
- Garum armoricum—fermented salted fish—is helpful for chronic fatigue, depression, and sleep problems.
- Use ginger to help arthritis.
- Some herbal supplements that help to induce sleep are ginseng, hops, kava kava, melatonin, passionflower, and valerian root.
- Horse chestnut helps strengthen veins and prevent leakage in varicose veins.
- Licorice, dong quai, and black cohosh are all herbs to help with hot flashes during menopause.
- Try taking a couple drops of peppermint oil on your tongue or in a small amount of water to help calm an upset or nervous stomach.
- Any man over fifty should consider taking the herb saw palmetto to keep the prostate from enlarging and help with the flow of urine.
- For increased sexual ability, six months of DHEA supplements will help. Also the amino acid arginine helps increase nitric oxide that is essential to a firm erection for men. Ginkgo biloba helps improve blood flow to the penis.
- Vitamin B1 (thiamine) taken daily during the summer will help ward off mosquitoes.

- If you are taking vitamin B12 tablets, it is best to do so sublingually (under the tongue).
- Willow bark helps mild pain disorders and lower back pain.

Therapy Facts

- Acupuncture may be used to help improve incontinence and manage pain.
- As help for Bursitis, try drinking water that has a squirt of liquid chlorophyll in it. Do this every day for a while and then, afterwards, repeat four or five times a week. Once, I could not lift my left arm above my shoulder without pain. Upon telling my herbalist, she said to follow the liquid chlorophyll procedure and the pain would move from my shoulder down to my elbow and then go away in two weeks. Sure enough, it worked.
- Many and maybe most heart attacks are caused by viral infections. CoQ10, magnesium, and vitamin E are primary ingredients to help fight a heart attack. Vitamin E is a strong antioxidant and is safe in reasonable doses. CoQ10 can help hypertension and angina. Magnesium, when taken along with potassium, helps the heart.
- Leg cramps can be dealt with by different treatments. The first way is stretching. If the calf of your leg tends to cramp, try standing with the ball of your foot and toes on a two- or three-inch-high object and let the heal of the foot extend down to touch the floor. By repeating this process two or three times for thirty seconds, your calf muscle will stretch and flexibility will increase. This should also help foot cramps, since the muscles are entwined. Magnesium is the second treatment, as it works as a muscle relaxant. Too much magnesium causes your colon muscles to relax and may give you loose stools. The third treatment is to take quinine water. Check to see if you are allergic to quinine before trying this method. Quinine sulfate capsules are available by prescription. The fourth treatment, if leg pain is consistent—which may be caused by blood flow blockages—can be helped by chelation therapy.
- Hair loss can be helped by the use of curetage (an all-natural) shampoo, conditioner, and scalp treatment. It helps stimulate the hair follicles to help hair growth.
- Weight training is a proven technique to improve muscle mass and strength. Care and assistance should be taken in starting a program.
- Thioctic acid will help clear metals from the tissues of your body.

- Some parasites and bacteria are asleep in our nervous system and only become active and aroused by stress.
- A gluten sensitivity test can tell if a person has an allergy to foods containing gluten, which can be the cause of a wide variety of symptoms including fatigue, joint aches, malaise, and thyroiditis.
- The pineal gland controls the levels of melatonin the body produces. Melatonin is often taken to help with sleep disorders. Melatonin levels in the blood, when elevated, can be a contributing factor for women with fibromyalgia and Chronic Fatigue Syndrome (CFS). The fact that women have larger pineal glands than men may be why women live longer. Melatonin might play a role in this scenario. Several popular drugs inhibit the body's production of melatonin.

CHAPTER 15
Author's Autobiography

Early Years

I was born at 11:34 PM on November 3, 1938, in Detroit, Michigan, U.S.A. and spent my early years living in the north edge of Detroit. I started playing baseball and working at a young age, had a paper route one summer for three months, and a job picking up golf balls at a driving range for two summers. My family moved to the suburbs, fourteen miles north of Detroit, half way through grade six. This was farm country, and I attended a one-room country school for a year and a half. Summers were spent working on the 120-acre farm next door or for another truck farmer down the road. I was bussed into town for grades eight through twelve. During my junior and senior years, evenings were spent sitting pins at the bowling alley after sports practice (baseball and basketball).

Teenage Years

After graduation, I went to Texas with eleven buddies from high school for basic training for the Michigan Air National Guard. I started college in September of 1956 for pre-dental education and lived at home. I worked the following summer at a gas station and then went back to college in September. I got expelled that year because I was caught drinking on campus at a party. I started working as a clerk at one of the local factories for a year and then went back to college in September of 1958 to study engineering. I lived on campus and worked the switchboard in the dorm. I had to pay tuition and room and board, in addition to reimbursing my father for my previous year's lost tuition. I tried out for the baseball team and made it, but not as a starter. I was not a good hitter.

Early Adult Years

I started working on June 30, 1959, in engineering and thought I had the world by the tail. I got married in 1960 and started raising a family. We bought a house with minimum down. I got laid off January 31, 1961, during a slow down, with new wife, new child, new house, and no money. This was very traumatic. After three months, I finally got another job as a clerk. This job lasted for five months until getting called back from the lay-off. I divorced my wife in 1968 and started paying child support for three sons.

Mid-life Experience

In 1970, I was working for a company as a design draftsman and got the chance to work in Sweden. It was a real opportunity to travel. There were six of us that went. I stayed in Sweden six months before choosing to leave because of possible income tax problems. I was in eleven countries in twenty-one days the first time I returned from Sweden in 1970. I returned to Sweden in 1971 for three more months, as the project still existed, and they wanted us to return.

Shortly after returning home from that trip, work got a little dicey; I had to move around from one job to another for a while. As it turns out, the company I was working for in 1974 was asked to give Volvo a quote for sending three employees back to Sweden. I found out that if you stayed out of the country working for more than twelve months, you would be eligible for a very large tax deduction. I stayed in Sweden for seventeen months with just one trip back to the states to load my automobile on a boat for shipment to Sweden.

Volvo closes down the entire month of July for vacations, so that summer I went to Scotland for a five-day trip. I met my wife on a bus trip and we have been happily married since June of 1977. We had many problems with immigration and finally had to go the fiancée-visa route, causing us to live in Windsor for three months while the visa was processed.

We had already rented an apartment, which was only ten minutes from my job; I commuted back and forth from Detroit to Windsor every day, while going to the apartment at lunchtime on an "as needed" basis to exchange clothes. Once the visa was issued, we had sixty days to get married.

We lived in the apartment for a year before buying a house. We lived there for twelve years. We wanted to move and found a dream place only three miles away. It was a great place on a man-made lake. We bartered on the asking price and finally reached an agreement. We made a deposit and put our house on the market. Things happened fast, and we moved into the new place with no prospects on our two-bedroom ranch.

We had to take a bridge loan to make the transition. The house on the lake had a couple large decks overlooking the water. It required a lot of upkeep, and since both my wife and I were working, we had to hire someone. After five years, we decided it was just too much and bought a new condo, where we presently live. I retired from work on June 30, 1999, after working forty years. The last fourteen years of my employment were spent working on a computer, so it was physically not as demanding. I am enjoying retirement.

References

The Zone by Barry Sears, Ph.D.

Into The Light by W.C. Douglass, M.D.

The Multiple Sclerosis Diet Book by Roy Swank, M.D., Ph.D. and Barbara Dugan

Forty-Something Forever by Arline & Harold Brecher

Oxygen Healing Therapies by Nathaniel Altman

Shaping Up With Vitamins by Earl Mindell, R.Ph., Ph.D.

Second Opinion monthly newsletter by William Campbell Douglas, M.D.

Health and Healing monthly newsletter by Julian Whitaker, M.D.

Hydrogen Peroxide Medical Miracle by WilliamCampbell Whitaker, M.D.

The Yeast Connection by William G. Crook, M.D.

Shaping Up with Vitamins by Earl Mindell

The Cure for all Diseases by Hulda Regehr Clark, Ph.D., N.D.

Nature's Choices by Julie Alkens

Prescription for Nutritional Healing by Phillis A. Balch, CNC and James F. Balch, M.D.

Appendix

Zapper Log (ref. Chapter 3)

QXCI Log (ref Chapter 3)

56 Reasons How Sugar Ruins your Health (ref. Chapter 4)

Reflexology Graphs (ref. Chapter 11)

Chakra Chart (ref. Chapter 11)

EDS Chart (ref. Chapter 12)

Hair Analysis (ref. Chapter 12)

Thermoscan Picture (ref. Chapter 12)

Zapper Log

09-23-00   Started "zapping."

09-24-00   Numbness in fingers was better and able to feel wood texture in door.

09-26-00   Tingling between shoulder and elbow was better.

09-30-00   Left ankle itched after I got in bed, previously not much feeling.

10-02-00   Wife commented it was easier for me to get out of bed.

10-03-00   Mobility and energy was better. Exercised one full hour.

10-08-00   Easier going up and down stairs using feet alternately.

10-12-00   Stood up straighter while brushing teeth and shaving.

10-19-00   Had itch on lower left leg.

10-20-00   Standing in shower washing and drying myself was better.

10-26-00   Stood up out of bed by pushing off bed, not grabbing on.

11-05-00   Traveled basement stairs better.

11-14-00   Increased energy and slept full night without having to get up.

11-17-00   Felt good and slept better. No nap in afternoon.

11-18-00   Pushed off bed to stand up.

11-28-00   Numbness in arms better and took a couple clumsy steps at PT.

12-01-00   Took two more steps at PT and two more at home to show my wife.

12-07-00   Eyesight seemed better and I had good energy.

12-15-00   Balance and coordination seemed slightly better.

12-17-00   Stood at side of bed to dress without support. Stood and hugged wife.

12-23-00   Felt stronger and seemed better walking with walker.

01-02-01   Was able to lift left knee up on chair to pick up something.

01-03-01   PT therapist said I was stronger and able to walk backwards better.

01-14-01   Crossed and un-crossed right leg over left knee without use of hands.

01-26-01   Coordination and ability to lean over improved slightly.

01-31-01   Coordination in shower was better.

02-01-01   After massage was able to go up stairs better.

02-05-01   Walking backwards at PT between parallel bars was easier.

02-06-01   Better agility in shower.

02-13-01   Coordination, energy, and left leg movement was better.

02-15-01   Tried movement in morning using tennis shoes and no AFO, not bad.

02-22-01   Good energy and mobility and forty-five minutes of exercise at PT.

03-05-01	Was wide-awake at 6:30 AM after going to bed at 10 PM previous night.
03-06-01	Better coordination while getting up during night.
03-26-01	Trip to doctor. Exacerbation and needed treatment.
03-27-01	Started solumedrol.
11-19-01	Pushed off bed to stand.
11-20-01	Was able to partially squat to pick something up and held on to stand.
11-23-01	Was able to walk a short way behind walker without holding on.
12-06-01	Noticed increased strength at PT and was able to move some furniture.
12-11-01	PT therapist commented on how noticeably stronger left leg was.
01-03-02	While sitting on chair, was able to raise right knee and extend foot.
01-04-02	From this day forward, I only used zapper occasionally.

QXCI Log

This is a record of treatments and improvements I have noticed while doing sessions on the QXCI machine

Chronological Progress

11-27-02	My first three-hour session. My benefits were: I buttoned my shirt, I did the stairs better, I stood while drying hands, I had more control of my right foot while driving, and I did not have to think about moving foot from throttle to brake.
11-30-02	I noticed the following: my balance was better standing in shower, when I stepped into my car my left leg just followed me in, and I was able to increase weights during exercise.
12-02-02	My second session, lasted 3.5 hours. My benefits were: I stood up from my chair by just pushing off the seat and rocking forward and I buttoned my shirt.
12-03-02	I rolled over in bed with more control during the night and stood with legs against the bed while dressing.
12-04-02	After my shower I was able to sit on a stool and dry feet without having to lean against the counter. I had better balance while dressing.
12-05-02	My third treatment lasted for two hours. My benefits were: climbing stairs into the house was better, I was able to get up from the sofa, and my eyesight seemed better.
12-06-03	I was able to stand better while pulling on pants and stood without holding on to blow dry hands after washing them.
12-07-02	I was almost able to sit up while getting out of bed, I had better finger control while cleaning razor, my wife said I was standing straighter, and I was able to push off and stand up from a chair on rollers.
12-10-02	My fourth session lasted for 2.5 hours. I was able to put on my coat while standing in the center of the room and pushed off and stood up from a folding chair.

12-11-03 I stood up much easier getting out of bed and I noticed I was lifting my left leg and bending the knee better.

12-13-02 My fifth session lasted for 3.5 hours. I was able to stretch out my left leg from underneath the emergency brake lever and I was able to lift my right leg from the throttle to the brake pedal.

12-16-02 I was able to bend both knees to lift my feet off the floor and I had more strength in my finger to work the alligator clips on my zapper.

12-17-02 My sixth session lasted for 2.5 hours. I picked up my walker and carried it for six steps.

12-18-02 At physical therapy, I had more strength and I rolled my left leg out of the driver's seat in my van without using my hands.

12-21-02 My seventh session lasted four hours. I was able to cross my right leg over my left leg.

01-03-03 My eighth session, for 2.5 hours.

01-07-03, 01-10-03, 01-15-03, 01-18-03, 01-22-03, 01-24-03, 01-29-03, 02-03-03, 2-05-03, 02-13-03, and 02-25-03

I had sessions, all for 2.5 to 3.5 hours. Minor improvements included movement on stairs and continued previous improvements.

03-07-03 I received my own QXCI machine and the healing process continues.

56 Reasons How Sugar Ruins Your Health

- Sugar may cause: (1) aging, (2) anxiety, (3) appendicitis, (4) arthritis, (5) asthma, (6) Candida Albicans, (7) cardiovascular disease, (8) cataracts, (9) changes in persons with gastric or duodenal ulcers, (10) changes in persons with functional bowel disease, (11) copper deficiency, (12) crankiness, (13) decrease in insulin sensitivity, (14) difficulty concentrating, (15) drowsiness, (16) food allergies, (17) free radicals in the blood stream, (18) emphysema, (19) gallstones, (20) heart disease, (21) hemorrhoids, (22) hyperactivity, (23) hypoglycemia, (24) kidney damage, (25) migraine headaches, (26) multiple sclerosis, (27) tooth decay, and (28) varicose veins.
- Sugar may contribute to: (29) diabetes, (30) eczema, (31) osteoporosis, (32) obesity, (33) reduction in defense against bacterial infections, and (34) saliva acidity.
- Sugar may decrease: (35) glucose tolerance and (36) growth hormones.
- Sugar may elevate (37) glucose and insulin responses in oral contraceptive users.
- Sugar may increase: (38) cholesterol, (39) fasting levels of glucose and insulin, (40) risk of Crohn's disease and ulcerative colitis, and (41) systolic blood pressure.
- Sugar may interfere with: (42) absorption of calcium and magnesium and (43) absorption of protein.
- Sugar may impair (44) the structure of DNA.
- Sugar may lead to: (45) alcoholism, (46) cancer of the breast, ovaries, intestines, prostate, rectum, and (47) chromium deficiency.
- Sugar may lower (48) the body's enzymes ability to function.
- Sugar may make (49) the skin age by changing the structure of collagen.
- Sugar may produce: (50) an acidic stomach and (51) a significant rise in triglycerides.
- Sugar may raise: (52) adrenaline levels and (53) the level of neurotransmitters called serotonin.
- Sugar may reduce (54) high-density lipoproteins (LDL).
- Sugar may suppress (55) the immune system.
- Sugar may upset (56) minerals in the body.

ReflexologyGraphs

Rainbow Coded Foot Reflexology Chart

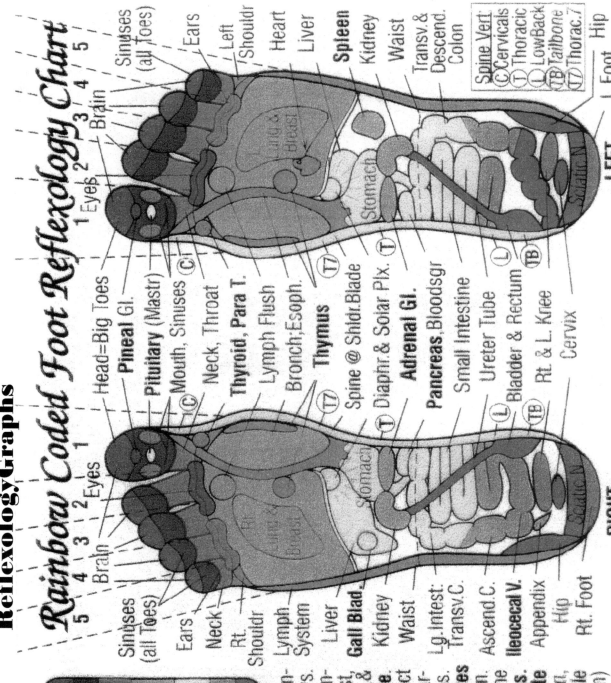

Head=Big Toes
Pineal Gl.
Pituitary (Mastr)
Mouth, Sinuses (C)
Neck, Throat
Thyroid, Para T.
Lymph Flush
Bronch;Esoph.
Thymus
Spine @ Shldr.Blade (T7)
Diaphr.& Solar Plx. (T)
Adrenal Gl.
Pancreas,Bloodsgr
Small Intestine
Ureter Tube (L)
Bladder & Rectum
Rt & L. Knee (TB)
Cervix

Sinuses (all Toes)
Ears
Neck
Rt. Shouldr
Lymph System
Liver
Gall Blad.
Kidney
Waist
Lg.Intest. Transv.C.
Ascend.C.
Ileocecal V.
Appendix
Hip
Rt. Foot
Sciatic N
RIGHT

Sinuses (all Toes)
Ears
Left Shouldr
Heart
Liver
Spleen
Kidney
Waist
Transv.& Descend. Colon

1 Eyes 2 3 Brain 4 5

5 4 3 2 Eyes 1
Brain

Spine Vert.
(C) Cervicals
(T) Thoracic
(L) LowBack
(TB) Tailbone
(T7) Thorac.7
L.Foot Hip
LEFT

Stomach

Reflexology helps rejuvinate our mental, emot.,& phys. well being + health by stimulating the circ. & nerv. Syst, healing, releasing tension,& increasing stress resilience. All points in our Ft. connect (via nerves,meridians)to particular organs & body areas.
Our Ft, Hands, Face, Eyes = the endpts. of 10 zones /en. channels.The 7 Colors = the 7 endocrine gls.+ 7 Chakras. Tenderness= calcium+ waste deposits frm preservs;caffein, alc;cigs, othr toxins + muscle acid (frm no exercise,tension) & /or illness in ea. area.

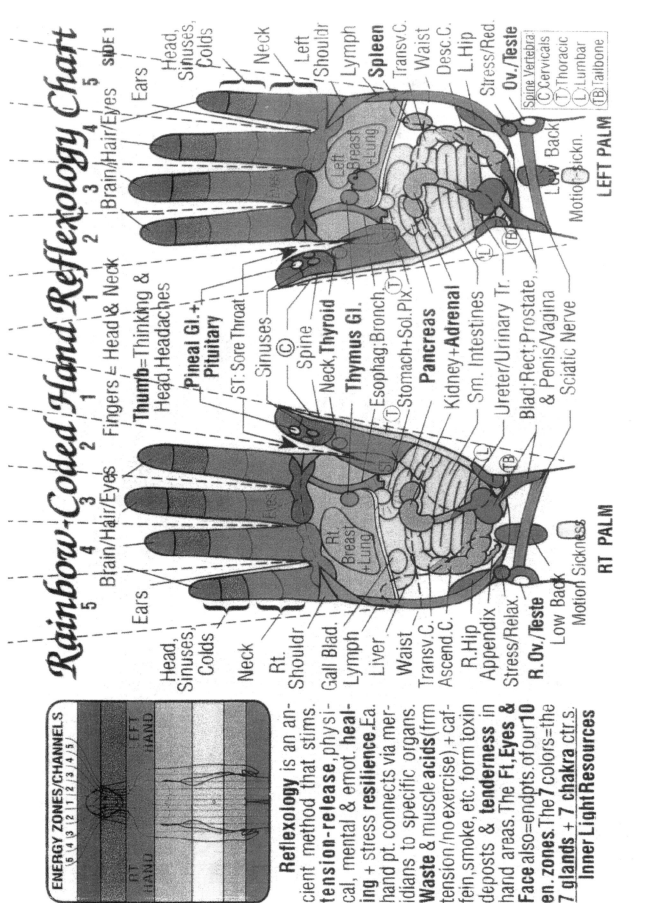

Rainbow+Coded Hand Reflexology Chart

SIDE 1

ENERGY ZONES/CHANNELS
5 4 3 2 1 1 2 3 4 5

RT HAND
LEFT HAND

RT PALM (right hand)

Fingers = Head & Neck

Thumb = Thinking & Head, Headaches

Pineal Gl. + Pituitary

ST: Sore Throat
Sinuses
Spine ©
Neck, **Thyroid**
Thymus Gl.
Esophag.; Bronch.
Stomach+Sol.Plx. (T)
Pancreas
Kidney+**Adrenal**
Sm. Intestines
Ureter/Urinary Tr.
Blad.;Rect;Prostate, & Penis/Vagina
Sciatic Nerve

Brain/Hair/Eyes 5 4 3
Ears
Head, Sinuses, Colds
Neck
Rt. Shouldr
Gall Blad.
Lymph
Liver
Waist
Transv.C.
Ascend.C.
R.Hip
Appendix
Stress/Relax.
R.Ov./Teste
Low Back
Motion Sickness

Rt. Breast +Lung

LEFT PALM

Brain/Hair/Eyes 2 3 4 5
Ears
Head, Sinuses, Colds
Neck
Left Shouldr
Lymph
Spleen
Transv.C.
Waist
Desc.C.
L.Hip
Stress/Red.
Ov./Teste
Low Back
Motion Sickn.

Left Breast +Lung

Spine Vertebra
© Cervicals
T Thoracic
L Lumbar
(TB) Tailbone

Reflexology is an ancient method that stims. **tension-release**, physical, mental & emot. **healing** + stress **resilience**. Ea. hand pt. connects via meridians to specific organs. **Waste** & muscle **acids** (frm tension/no exercise),+ caffein,smoke, etc. form toxin deposts & **tenderness** in hand areas. The **Ft,Eyes & Face** also=endpts.of our **10 en. zones**. The **7** colors=the **7 glands + 7 chakra** ctr.s.

Inner Light Resources

Chakra Chart

Chakra #	Color	Purpose	Orientation to self	Glands & organs, connections	Connection to emotional and mental	Connection to physical body	Element related	Excessive characteristic	Deficient characteristic
1 - Root Base of spine	Red & black	Energy, grounding. survival	Self preservation	Adrenals, bones, colon, feet, kidneys, spinal column	Family, safety, security	Low back, rectal area, sciatica, veins	Earth	Greed, materialism, monotony, sluggish	Fear, no discipline, restless, spacey
2 - Sacral Abdomen Genitals	Orange	Digestion Emotions, Sexuality	Self gratification	Bladder, ovaries, prostate, spleen, testicles	Blame, control, guilt, money, power, sex	Bladder, pelvic, potency, urinary	Water	addiction, behavior, emotional, obsessive, sex	Frigidity, impotence, numbness, rigidity
3 - Solar Plexus	Yellow	Ego, intellectual, self interest, will power	Self definition	Gallbladder, liver, pancreas, stomach, upper intestine	Honor, respect, self-esteem, trust	Anorexia, arthritis, diabetes, hepatitis	Fire	Aggressive, blaming, dominating, very active	Fearful, low esteem passive, weak will
4 - Heart	Green & pink	Anger, hate, love, relationships	Self acceptance	Arms, lungs, circulation, diaphragm, hands, heart, ribs, thymus	Anger, grief, hate, love, loneliness, resentment	Allergies, asthma, cancer, lung, circulation	Air	Codependency, jealous, possessive	Bitter, critical, lonely, shy
5 -Throat	Blue	Communication, expression, speech	Self expression	Gums, neck, mouth, parathyroid, teeth, throat	Addiction, decisions, dreams, faith, knowledge	Depression, Joint problems, laryngitis	Sound	Inability to listen stuttering, talkative	Fear of speaking poor rhythm, quiet
6 - Brow	Indigo	Fear, insight, imagination, inspiration, intuition, thought	Self reflection	Brain, eyes, ears, nervous system, nose, pineal, pituitary	Abilities, feelings, openness, truth	Blindness, deafness, neurological, stroke, tumors	Light	Delusions, hallucinations, headaches, nightmares,	Denial, poor vision & memory
7 - Crown	Violet	Awareness, central nervous system, hormones, skin	Self knowledge	Cerebral Cortex muscular & skeletal systems	Courage, devotion, selflessness, spirituality, trust, values	Depression, fatigue, sensitivity	Information	Confusion, dissociation, intellectual, spiritual	Apathy, learning difficulty materialism, skeptic

EDS Chart

Items Tested	Dilution	Point ID	Max	Drop	
Info-Sensitivity Screening by Groups\Food					
1. Dairy	Stress Test	NE-1b*R	67	0	
2. Additives	Stress Test	NE-1b*R	63	0	
3. Grains	Stress Test	NE-1b*R	63	0	
4. Dairy	Stress Test	NE-1b*R	62	1	
5. International Foods	Stress Test	NE-1b*R	61	1	
6. Nuts - Seeds	Stress Test	NE-1b*R	60	1	
7. Additives	Stress Test	NE-1b*R	59	1	
8. Dairy	Stress Test	NE-1b*R	58	0	
9. Dairy	Stress Test	NE-1b*R	58	0	
10. Meat - Poultry	Stress Test	NE-1b*R	56	0	
11. Spices	Stress Test	NE-1b*R	56	0	
12. Vegetables	Stress Test	NE-1b*R	55	0	
13. Legumes - Beans	Stress Test	NE-1b*R	54	0	
14. Fish	Stress Test	NE-1b*R	54	0	
15. Fruit	Stress Test	NE-1b*R	54	0	
16. Shellfish	Stress Test	NE-1b*R	53	0	
17. Beverages	Stress Test	NE-1b*R	52	0	
18. Fish	Stress Test	NE-1b*R	52	0	
19. Condiments	Stress Test	NE-1b*R	52	0	
20. Sugars & Sweeteners	Stress Test	NE-1b*R	52	0	
21. Supplements	Stress Test	NE-1b*R	51	0	
22. Cooking Oils	Stress Test	NE-1b*R	50	0	
23. Baking & Cooking Ingredients	Stress Test	NE-1b*R	49	0	
Info-Sensitivity Screening by Groups\Food\Additives					
24. Monosodium Glutamate (MSG)	Stress Test	NE-1b*R	68	0	
25. Butylated Hydroxytoluene (BHT)	Stress Test	NE-1b*R	67	0	
26. Dye, Red	Stress Test	NE-1b*R	66	1	
27. Dye, Blue	Stress Test	NE-1b*R	66	0	
28. Chlorine	Stress Test	NE-1b*R	63	0	
29. Sodium Nitrite	Stress Test	NE-1b*R	62	0	
30. Butylated Hydroxyanisole (BHA)	Stress Test	NE-1b*R	61	1	
31. Dye, Yellow	Stress Test	NE-1b*R	61	0	

Weakened   Balanced   Stressed

32. Calcium Sorbate	Stress Test	NE-1b*R	58	2	
33. Maltol	Stress Test	NE-1b*R	58	0	
34. Acid benzoicum	Stress Test	NE-1b*R	58	0	
35. Lecithin	Stress Test	NE-1b*R	58	1	
36. Hydrolyzed Vegetable Protein	Stress Test	NE-1b*R	58	0	
37. Vitamin E	Stress Test	NE-1b*R	57	0	
38. Glycerine, Animal	Stress Test	NE-1b*R	57	0	
39. Guar Bean	Stress Test	NE-1b*R	57	0	
40. Alginic Acid	Stress Test	NE-1b*R	56	0	
41. Acid sorbicum	Stress Test	NE-1b*R	55	0	
42. Carageenan	Stress Test	NE-1b*R	54	0	
43. Agar Agar	Stress Test	NE-1b*R	54	0	
44. Riboflavin	Stress Test	NE-1b*R	54	0	
45. Sodium Nitrate	Stress Test	NE-1b*R	54	0	
46. Sodium Metabisulfite	Stress Test	NE-1b*R	54	0	
47. Gum, Tragacanth	Stress Test	NE-1b*R	54	0	
48. Gum, Karaya (Basorum)	Stress Test	NE-1b*R	54	0	
49. Gum, Acacia (Arabic)	Stress Test	NE-1b*R	53	0	
50. Saffron	Stress Test	NE-1b*R	52	0	
51. Tartrazine	Stress Test	NE-1b*R	52	1	
52. Sorbic Acid	Stress Test	NE-1b*R	52	0	
53. Sodium Sulfate	Stress Test	NE-1b*R	52	0	
54. Sodium Fluoride	Stress Test	NE-1b*R	52	0	
55. Turmeric	Stress Test	NE-1b*R	52	1	
56. Glycerine, Vegetable	Stress Test	NE-1b*R	51	0	
57. Na-o-phenylphenolat	Stress Test	NE-1b*R	50	0	
58. Vitamin C	Stress Test	NE-1b*R	50	0	
59. Sulfur Dioxide	Stress Test	NE-1b*R	50	0	
60. Xanthan Gum	Stress Test	NE-1b*R	48	0	
61. Pectin	Stress Test	NE-1b*R	48	0	

Info-Sensitivity Screening by Groups\Food\Dairy

62. Cheese - Feta	Stress Test	NE-1b*R	68	0	
63. Lactose	Stress Test	NE-1b*R	67	0	
64. Albumin, Cowmilk	Stress Test	NE-1b*R	67	0	
65. Cheese - Cottage	Stress Test	NE-1b*R	66	0	
66. Cheese - Cheddar	Stress Test	NE-1b*R	66	0	
67. Butter	Stress Test	NE-1b*R	65	1	
68. Cheese - Cream	Stress Test	NE-1b*R	64	0	
69. Cheese - Swiss	Stress Test	NE-1b*R	64	0	
70. Cheese - American	Stress Test	NE-1b*R	64	0	
71. Casein - Cow	Stress Test	NE-1b*R	63	0	
72. Cheese - Parmesan	Stress Test	NE-1b*R	63	0	
73. Cheese - Camembert	Stress Test	NE-1b*R	63	0	
74. Cheese - Roquefort	Stress Test	NE-1b*R	63	0	
75. Cheese - Mozzarella	Stress Test	NE-1b*R	63	0	
76. Whey - Cow	Stress Test	NE-1b*R	63	0	
77. Cheese - Sheep	Stress Test	NE-1b*R	62	0	
78. Cheese - Romano	Stress Test	NE-1b*R	62	0	
79. Cream	Stress Test	NE-1b*R	62	0	
80. Milk - Raw	Stress Test	NE-1b*R	61	2	
81. Cheese - Muenster	Stress Test	NE-1b*R	57	0	
82. Milk - Pastuerized	Stress Test	NE-1b*R	57	0	
83. Kefir	Stress Test	NE-1b*R	56	0	
84. Milk - Goat	Stress Test	NE-1b*R	56	0	

☐ Weakened	▨ Balanced	■ Stressed

85. Margarine	Stress Test	NE-1b*R	55	0	
86. Milk - Almond	Stress Test	NE-1b*R	55	0	
87. Egg - Yolk	Stress Test	NE-1b*R	54	0	
88. Milk - Cow	Stress Test	NE-1b*R	54	0	
89. Egg - Whole	Stress Test	NE-1b*R	52	0	
90. Yoghurt - Cow	Stress Test	NE-1b*R	52	1	
91. Cheese - Goat	Stress Test	NE-1b*R	51	0	
92. Milk - Sheep	Stress Test	NE-1b*R	51	0	
93. Egg - White	Stress Test	NE-1b*R	50	0	
94. Milk - Soya	Stress Test	NE-1b*R	49	1	
95. Yoghurt - Sheep	Stress Test	NE-1b*R	49	0	
96. Milk - Rice	Stress Test	NE-1b*R	47	1	

Info-Sensitivity Screening by Groups\Food\Grains

97. Wheat, Organic	Stress Test	NE-1b*R	66	3	
98. Wheat, White Flour	Stress Test	NE-1b*R	64	0	
99. Amaranth	Stress Test	NE-1b*R	62	0	
100. Wheat Germ	Stress Test	NE-1b*R	61	0	
101. Wheat - Whole	Stress Test	NE-1b*R	61	0	
102. Gliadin	Stress Test	NE-1b*R	58	1	
103. Rye	Stress Test	NE-1b*R	58	0	
104. Kamut	Stress Test	NE-1b*R	57	0	
105. Corn - White	Stress Test	NE-1b*R	57	0	
106. Rice	Stress Test	NE-1b*R	56	1	
107. Corn	Stress Test	NE-1b*R	55	0	
108. Corn - Blue	Stress Test	NE-1b*R	55	0	
109. Wheat - Bran	Stress Test	NE-1b*R	54	0	
110. Millet	Stress Test	NE-1b*R	54	0	
111. Rice, Bran	Stress Test	NE-1b*R	54	0	
112. Wild Rice	Stress Test	NE-1b*R	54	0	
113. Corn - Red	Stress Test	NE-1b*R	54	0	
114. Corn - Yellow	Stress Test	NE-1b*R	54	0	
115. Quinoa	Stress Test	NE-1b*R	53	0	
116. Oat	Stress Test	NE-1b*R	52	0	
117. Popcorn	Stress Test	NE-1b*R	52	0	
118. Teff	Stress Test	NE-1b*R	51	0	
119. Gluten	Stress Test	NE-1b*R	51	1	
120. Barley	Stress Test	NE-1b*R	50	0	
121. Spelt	Stress Test	NE-1b*R	50	0	
122. Buckwheat	Stress Test	NE-1b*R	50	0	

	Weakened		Balanced		Stressed

Base Readings

Point ID	Meridian	Max	Min	Rise	Fall	Drop	
LY-1R	Lymphatics	50	48	38	2	2	
LY-1-1R	Lymphatics	52	52	45	0	0	
LY-1-2*R	Lymphatics	66	65	51	0	1	
LY-2R	Lymphatics	53	53	56	0	0	
LY-3R	Lymphatics	52	51	29	0	1	
LU-10c*R	Lungs	48	48	36	0	0	
LI-1b*R	Large Intestine	48	48	26	0	0	
NE-1b*R	Nervous System	50	48	20	3	2	
CI-8d*R	Circulation	48	48	52	0	0	
AL-1R	Allergies	65	64	54	0	1	
AL-1b*R	Allergies	61	61	40	0	0	
OR-1b*R	Cellular Metabolism	49	49	37	0	0	
TW-1R	Endocrine System	56	56	35	0	0	
TW-1b*R	Endocrine System	61	60	50	0	1	
TW-2R	Endocrine System	52	49	31	6	3	
TW-3R	Endocrine System	53	53	27	0	0	
HE-8c*R	Heart	50	50	32	0	0	
SI-1b*R	Small Intestine	51	51	29	0	0	
SI-3*R	Small Intestine	52	51	37	0	1	
LY-1L	Lymphatics	51	49	34	3	2	
LY-1-1L	Lymphatics	53	50	49	6	3	
LY-1-2*L	Lymphatics	54	53	36	0	1	
LY-2L	Lymphatics	55	55	35	0	0	
LY-3L	Lymphatics	55	55	55	0	0	
LU-10c*L	Lungs	50	49	41	0	1	
LI-1b*L	Large Intestine	49	49	30	0	0	
NE-1b*L	Nervous System	60	60	50	0	0	
CI-8d*L	Circulation	48	47	36	0	1	
AL-1L	Allergies	70	67	58	4	3	
AL-1b*L	Allergies	64	64	35	0	0	
OR-1b*L	Cellular Metabolism	54	54	40	0	0	
TW-1L	Endocrine System	52	52	46	0	0	
TW-1b*L	Endocrine System	54	53	56	0	1	
TW-2L	Endocrine System	52	49	38	4	3	
TW-3L	Endocrine System	50	50	23	0	0	
SI-3*L	Small Intestine	49	49	36	0	0	

Weakened   Balanced   Stressed

NUTRIENT MINERALS

	Ca	Mg	Na	K	Cu	Zn	P	Fe	Mn	Cr	Se	B	Co	Ge	Mo	Si	S	V
	Calcium	Magnesium	Sodium	Potassium	Copper	Zinc	Phosphorus	Iron	Manganese	Chromium	Selenium	Boron	Cobalt	Germanium	Molybdenum	Silicon	Sulfur	Vanadium
Current	18	3	5	2	1.2	19	15	.6	.01	.01	.07	.23	.002	.02	.002	N/A	4524	.002
Previous	27	4	4	3	.8	15	13	1.1	.01	.01	.02	.20	.002	.02	.002	.02	3989	.002

TOXIC MINERALS

	As	Be	Hg	Cd	Pb	Al
	Arsenic	Beryllium	Mercury	Cadmium	Lead	Aluminum
Current	.03	.002	.01	.01	.1	.3
Previous	.02	.002	.02	.01	.1	.5

ADDITIONAL MINERALS

	Sb	Ba	Bi	Au	Li	Ni	Pt	Ru	Sc	Ag	Sr	Sn	Ti	W	Zr
	Antimony	Barium	Bismuth	Gold	Lithium	Nickel	Platinum	Ruthenium	Scandium	Silver	Strontium	Tin	Titanium	Tungsten	Zirconium
Current	.03	.02	N/A	.02	.002	.1	.02	N/A	N/A	.01	.02	.02	.06	.04	.02
Previous	.02	.02	N/A	.02	.002	.1	.01	N/A	N/A	.01	.03	.02	.10	.04	.03

" << ": Below Calibration Limit; Value Given is Calibration Limit.

"QNS": Sample Size Was Inadequate For Analysis.

"NA": Currently Not Available

All Mineral Levels Are Reported in Mg%. (Milligrams Per One-Hundred Grams of Hair)

Ideal Levels And Interpretation Have Been Based On Hair Samples Obtained From The Mid-Parietal To The Occipital Region Of The Scalp.

Laboratory Analysis Provided By Trace Elements, Inc., an H.H.S. Licensed Clinical Laboratory. No. 45 D0481787

05/22/96
CURRENT TEST RESULTS

04/24/95
PREVIOUS TEST RESULTS

NUTRIENT MINERALS

TOXIC MINERALS

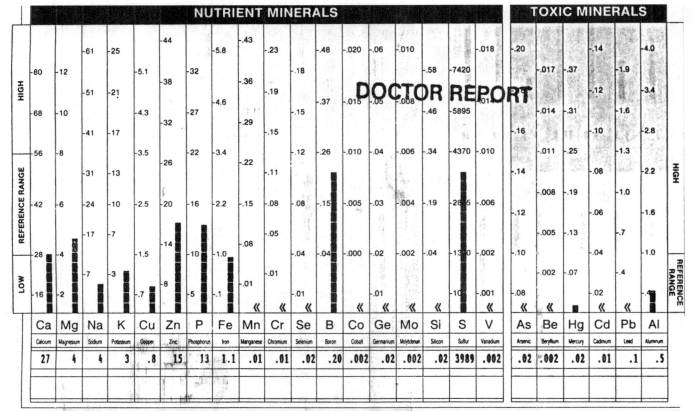

DOCTOR REPORT

	Ca	Mg	Na	K	Cu	Zn	P	Fe	Mn	Cr	Se	B	Co	Ge	Mo	Si	S	V	As	Be	Hg	Cd	Pb	Al
	Calcium	Magnesium	Sodium	Potassium	Copper	Zinc	Phosphorus	Iron	Manganese	Chromium	Selenium	Boron	Cobalt	Germanium	Molybdenum	Silicon	Sulfur	Vanadium	Arsenic	Beryllium	Mercury	Cadmium	Lead	Aluminum
	27	4	4	3	.8	15	13	1.1	.01	.01	.02	.20	.002	.02	.002	.02	3989	.002	.02	.002	.02	.01	.1	.5

ADDITIONAL MINERALS

	Sb	Ba	Bi	Au	Li	Ni	Pt	Ru	Sc	Ag	Sr	Sn	Ti	W	Zr
	Antimony	Barium	Bismuth	Gold	Lithium	Nickel	Platinum	Ruthenium	Scandium	Silver	Strontium	Tin	Titanium	Tungsten	Zirconium
	.02	.02	N/A	.02	.002	.1	.01	N/A	N/A	.01	.03	.02	.10	.04	.03

" << ": Below Calibration Limit; Value Given is Calibration Limit.

"QNS": Sample Size Was Inadequate For Analysis.

"NA": Currently Not Available

All Mineral Levels Are Reported in Mg%. (Milligrams Per One-Hundred Grams of Hair)

Ideal Levels And Interpretation Have Been Based On Hair Samples Obtained From The Mid-Parietal To The Occipital Region Of The Scalp.

Laboratory Analysis Provided By Trace Elements, Inc., an H.H.S. Licensed Clinical Laboratory. No. 45 D0481787

04/24/95
CURRENT TEST RESULTS

PREVIOUS TEST RESULTS

Hair Analysis Chart

POTENTIALLY TOXIC ELEMENTS

TOXIC ELEMENTS	RESULT μg/g	REFERENCE RANGE	PERCENTILE 68th	95th
Aluminum	36	< 7.0		
Antimony	0.15	< 0.066		
Arsenic	0.086	< 0.08		
Beryllium	< 0.01	< 0.02		
Bismuth	0.019	< 0.06		
Cadmium	0.088	< 0.15		
Lead	0.3	< 2.0		
Mercury	1.1	< 1.1		
Platinum	< 0.003	< 0.005		
Thallium	< 0.001	< 0.01		
Thorium	0.001	< 0.005		
Uranium	0.008	< 0.06		
Nickel	0.14	< 0.4		
Silver	0.04	< 0.12		
Tin	0.4	< 0.3		
Titanium	3.7	< 1.0		
Total Toxic Representation				

ESSENTIAL AND OTHER ELEMENTS

ELEMENTS	RESULT μg/g	REFERENCE RANGE	PERCENTILE 2.5th	16th	50th	84th	97.5th
Calcium	410	200- 750					
Magnesium	70	25- 75					
Sodium	69	12- 90					
Potassium	14	9.0- 40					
Copper	12	10- 28					
Zinc	240	130- 200					
Manganese	0.95	0.15- 0.65					
Chromium	1.6	0.2- 0.4					
Vanadium	0.027	0.018- 0.065					
Molybdenum	0.032	0.025- 0.064					
Boron	3.7	0.4- 3.0					
Iodine	0.39	0.25- 1.3					
Lithium	0.015	0.007- 0.023					
Phosphorus	330	160- 250					
Selenium	1.5	0.95- 1.7					
Strontium	0.96	0.3- 3.5					
Sulfur	50800	44500- 52000					
Barium	0.38	0.16- 1.6					
Cobalt	0.017	0.013- 0.035					
Iron	19	5.4- 13					
Germanium	0.037	0.045- 0.065					
Rubidium	0.028	0.011- 0.12					
Zirconium	1.3	0.02- 0.44					

SPECIMEN DATA

COMMENTS:

Date Collected: 3/11/2003
Date Received: 3/15/2003
Date Completed: 3/17/2003

Methodology: ICP-MS

Sample Size: 0.204 g
Sample Type: Head
Hair Color: Brown
Treatment:
Shampoo: White Rian

V06.99

RATIOS

ELEMENTS	RATIOS	EXPECTED RANGE
Ca/Mg	5.86	4- 30
Ca/P	1.24	0.8- 8
Na/K	4.93	0.5- 10
Zn/Cu	20	4- 20
Zn/Cd	> 999	> 800

Thermoscan Picture

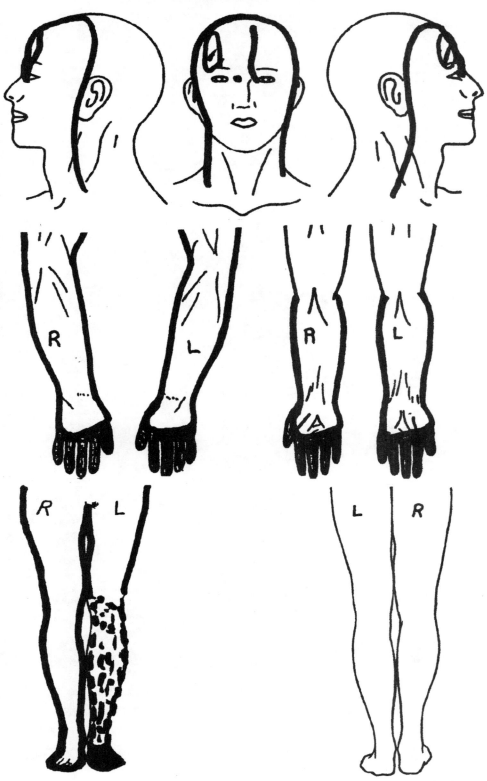